Dx/Rx:

Head and Neck Cancer

Kenneth S. Hu, MD
Department of Radiation Oncology
Beth Israel Hospital
New York, New York

Robert I. Haddad, MD
Department of Medical Oncology
Dana-Farber Cancer Institute
Boston, Massachusetts

Adam Jacobson, MD
Department of Otolaryngology – Head and Neck Surgery
Beth Israel Hospital
Albert Einstein College of Medicine
New York, New York

Series Editor: Manish A. Shah, MD
Director of Gastrointestinal Oncology
Weill Cornell Medical College/New-York-Presbyterian
Hospital
New York, New York

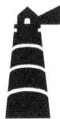

JONES & BARTLETT
L E A R N I N G

World Headquarters
Jones & Bartlett Learning
5 Wall Street
Burlington, MA 01803
978-443-5000
info@jblearning.com
www.jblearning.com

Jones & Bartlett Learning Canada
6339 Ormindale Way
Mississauga, Ontario L5V 1J2
Canada

Jones & Bartlett Learning International
Barb House, Barb Mews
London W6 7PA
United Kingdom

Jones & Bartlett Learning books and products are available through most bookstores and
online booksellers. To contact Jones & Bartlett Learning directly, call 800-832-0034, fax
978-443-8000, or visit our website, www.jblearning.com.

Substantial discounts on bulk quantities of Jones & Bartlett Learning publications are available
to corporations, professional associations, and other qualified organizations. For details and
specific discount information, contact the special sales department at Jones & Bartlett Learning
via the above contact information or send an email to specialsales@jblearning.com.

The authors, editor, and publisher have made every effort to provide accurate information.
However, they are not responsible for errors, omissions, or for any outcomes related to
the use of the contents of this book and take no responsibility for the use of the products
and procedures described. Treatments and side effects described in this book may not be
applicable to all people; likewise, some people may require a dose or experience a side
effect that is not described herein. Drugs and medical devices are discussed that may have
limited availability controlled by the Food and Drug Administration (FDA) for use only in a
research study or clinical trial. Research, clinical practice, and government regulations often
change the accepted standard in this field. When consideration is being given to use of any
drug in the clinical setting, the healthcare provider or reader is responsible for determining
FDA status of the drug, reading the package insert, and reviewing prescribing information
for the most up-to-date recommendations on dose, precautions, and contraindications, and
determining the appropriate usage for the product. This is especially important in the case
of drugs that are new or seldom used.

Production Credits
Executive Publisher: Christopher Davis
Associate Editor: Laura Burns
Associate Production Editor: Jill Morton
Associate Marketing Manager:
    Katie Hennessy
Manufacturing and Inventory Control
    Supervisor: Amy Bacus

Composition: Cenveo Publisher Services
Cover Design: Kate Ternullo
Cover Image: © LiquidLibrary
Printing and Binding: Malloy Incorporated
Cover Printing: Malloy Incorporated

Some images in this book feature models. These models do not necessarily endorse,
represent, or participate in the activities represented in the images.

Library of Congress Cataloging-in-Publication Data

Hu, Kenneth.
    Dx/Rx. Head and neck cancer / Kenneth S. Hu, Robert I. Haddad, Adam Jacobson.
        p. ; cm. -- (Dx/Rx oncology series)
    Head and neck cancer
    Includes bibliographical references and index.
    ISBN-13: 978-0-7637-8165-1
    ISBN-10: 0-7637-8165-7
    1. Head—Cancer—Treatment—Handbooks, manuals, etc. 2. Neck—Cancer—Treatment—
Handbooks, manuals, etc. I. Haddad, Robert I. II. Jacobson, Adam. III. Title. IV. Title: Head
and neck cancer. V. Series: Jones and Bartlett Publishers Dx/Rx oncology series.
    [DNLM: 1. Head and Neck Neoplasms—therapy—Handbooks. 2. Head and Neck
Neoplasms—diagnosis—Handbooks. WE 39]
    RC280.H4H8 2012
    616.99'491--dc23
                                            2011024629
6048

Printed in the United States of America
15 14 13 12 11 10 9 8 7 6 5 4 3 2 1

Contents

Editor's Preface

Welcome to the Dx/Rx Oncology Series. This current addition, Dx/Rx: *Head and Neck Cancer*, written by Drs. Hu, Haddad, and Jacobson, is an exceptional volume covering a broad and complex range of malignancies of the head and neck. As is true of all volumes in the Dx/Rx Oncology Series, this text is easy to read with to-the-point bullets, key data tables, and figures to allow for quick access to critical information for the diagnosis and management of disease. This particular volume is well organized with key chapters covering distinct types of head and neck malignancies including oral cavity, oropharynx, hypopharynx/larynx, and nasopharyngeal tumors. Furthermore, the text very eloquently highlights the multidisciplinary management of these diseases including the indications for surgery, radiation, or chemoradiation. Overall, you will find this text to be an invaluable resource in the management of the complex malignancies of the head and neck.

Manish A. Shah, MD

Preface

Head and neck carcinoma is the fourth most common cancer in the world, affecting close to half a million individuals each year. The main causes of head and neck cancer are smoking/chewing tobacco products, excessive alcohol use, and viral infection with human papilloma virus (HPV) or Epstein-Barr virus (EBV). A diagnosis of head and neck cancer has major implications with regard to quality of life because of the profound impact of a cancer originating in this area on a person's appearance, speech, swallowing, and breathing, as well as their ability to socially interact. Head and neck cancer is not "one disease" but comprises a large constellation of various subsites, and each has a particular pattern of spread that may require multimodality treatment and has different implications for cosmesis and function. A larynx cancer, for example, can require a simple laser excision or may require multiple courses of chemotherapy combined with two months of radiation.

The treatment of head and neck cancer is fairly complex, and significant expertise is required to manage these patients. A patient with a head and neck cancer typically requires evaluation by multiple specialists including a head and neck surgeon, medical oncologist, radiation oncologist, head and neck reconstructive surgeon, dentist, speech and swallowing therapist, dietician, nurse, social worker, physical therapist, and pain specialist. Yet, such an assembly of qualified individuals is rarely available at a single institution, making the management of these patients quite challenging.

The surgical management of head and neck cancer has evolved dramatically over the recent years because of the major advances made in head and neck reconstructive surgery. The ability to transfer tissue with high reliability has allowed ablative surgeons to approach tumors that were once thought to be insurmountable. Contemporary head and neck reconstructive techniques have allowed surgeons to restore both form and function to patients who in the past would have been left functionally and socially crippled.

Multiple techniques of radiation that precisely target the tumor and spare normal tissue are now available and can be very effective when used in the proper circumstance. Understanding how to treat the tumor and where it may potentially spread, while preserving the function of adjacent organs, becomes critical in helping a patient cure their cancer and maintain their quality of life.

Novel chemotherapy and biologic treatments, advances in functional imaging, and molecular understanding of the disease are constantly evolving, but understanding these advancements remains a daunting task for patients and caregivers. An example is the recent identification of HPV as a major cause of head and neck cancer in the western world. This has major implications for prognosis and potentially treatment of patients. A clear shift in the epidemiology of this disease is occurring because of this finding.

This book is written from a multidisciplinary perspective to increase awareness among healthcare and allied professionals who may encounter head and neck cancer patients. This text addresses the current, state-of-the-art management paradigms so that insights may be gleaned to better understand the sometimes overwhelming experience patients undergo and help them recover optimally. Too often head and neck cancer is just pigeon-holed as a black-box topic that is too difficult to understand. It is our hope that this text will shed more light on a cancer, for which major strides have been made to increase cure rates, function preservation, and quality of life.

Kenneth S. Hu, MD
Robert I. Haddad, MD
Adam Jacobson, MD

Acknowledgments and Dedications

To my family, teachers, colleagues, and patients who have made possible a highly rewarding and personally gratifying career in such a fascinating area of oncology. It is wonderful to make a difference in another person's well being and witness their transition from a cancer patient back to their place in society and family.

Kenneth S. Hu, MD

To my patients and their families, your daily fight against cancer and your courage is a source of inspiration to all of us.

My wife, Pascale, your love and support is truly unbelievable. You are my hero.

To Kelly Mia and Elsa Maria, my two wonderful daughters. You bring joy to my life every single day.

Robert I. Haddad, MD

To my wife, Marina, you are my inspiration.

To my three amazing daughters, you bring happiness and excitement to my life in ways that I could never have imagined.

To my patients and their families, you are the true heroes in our fight against cancer.

Adam Jacobson, MD

Notice

We have made every attempt to summarize accurately and concisely a multitude of references. However, the reader is reminded that times and medical knowledge change, transcription or understanding error is always possible, and crucial details can be omitted whenever such a comprehensive distillation as this is attempted in limited space. The primary purpose of this compilation is to cite literature on various sides of controversial issues; knowing where truth lies is usually difficult. We cannot, therefore, guarantee that every bit of information is absolutely accurate or complete. The reader should affirm that cited recommendations are reasonable still by reading the original articles and checking other sources, including local consultants as well as recent literature, before applying them.

Drugs and medical devices that may have limited availability controlled by the Food and Drug Administration (FDA) for use only in research study or clinical trial are discussed. The drug information presented has been derived from reference sources, recently published data, and pharmaceutical tests. Research, clinical practice, and government regulations often change the accepted standard in this field. When consideration is being given to use of any drug in the clinical setting, the clinician or reader is responsible for determining FDA status of the drug, reading the package insert, and prescribing information for the most up-to-date recommendations on dose, precautions, and contraindications and determining the appropriate usage for the product. This is especially important in the case of drugs that are new or seldom used.

General Principles of Treatment Approaches and Techniques for Head and Neck Squamous Cell Cancer

■ Introduction

- About 48,000 cases of head and neck cancer are diagnosed annually in United States.
- Squamous cell carcinoma is the histology in 95%.
- Fewer than 5% comprise lymphoma, minor salivary gland, melanoma, sarcoma, or plasmacytoma.
- Risk factors include alcohol, tobacco use, viral infections (human papilloma virus and Epstein-Barr virus), and betel nut chewing.
- One third present as stage I and II (node-negative small tumors).
- Two thirds present as stage III and IV (node-positive or large tumors).

■ Signs and Symptoms

- Throat or ear pain, hoarseness, dyspnea, difficulty swallowing, trismus, painless neck node, cranial neuropathy, stridor, and tongue fixation.

■ Workup/Staging

- History with attention to smoking history, risk factors for human papilloma virus and physical with focus on visualization and palpation of tumor site and cervical nodes,

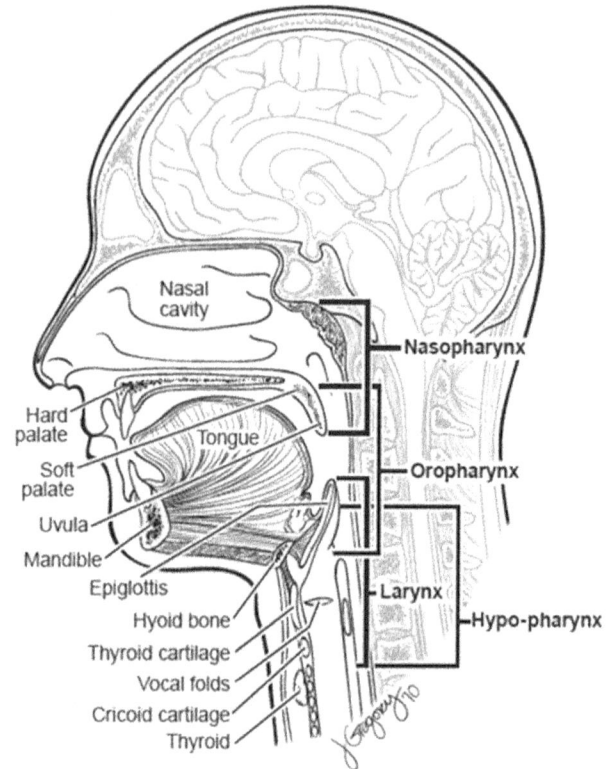

Figure 1.1 Anatomy of the Head and Neck Illustrating Common Mucosal Sites from Which Squamous Cell Carcinomas May Originate.

Note the intimate relationship of organs important for articulation, phonation, swallowing, and breathing.
Source: Courtesy of Jill K. Gregory, Continuum Health Partners.

assessment for extent of involvement of adjacent structures, and surveillance for a metachronous primary of the aerodigestive tract.

- Fiber-optic examination to evaluate areas not readily visualized on direct physical exam, such as tongue base, larynx, hypopharynx, nasopharynx, and nasal cavity.
- Examination under anesthesia for thorough palpation, biopsy, and comprehensive evaluation of aerodigestive tract.

- Computed tomography scan with contrast of neck to evaluate the initial lesion and regional spread including soft tissue and bony involvement.
- Magnetic resonance imaging with and without contrast is more accurate for soft-tissue delineation particularly for tumors with high predilection for perineural spread or intracranial or orbital invasion, and it can also distinguish between mucus secretions and tumor.
- Ultrasound may be used to assess neck masses.
- Positron-emission tomography/computed tomography scans to assess nodal involvement and rule out distant metastasis. A 3-month posttreatment scan can evaluate for persistent disease and determine if a salvage surgery is needed.
- Multidisciplinary pretreatment evaluation by
  - Surgeon, radiation oncologist, and medical oncologists.
  - Allied professionals, such as nurses, dentists, nutritionists, social workers, speech and swallowing therapists, and psychologists.
    - Preradiation dental consultation with panoramic x-ray imaging, dental extractions if indicated, and fluoride trays.
    - Speech and swallowing therapists are important to evaluate baseline function as well as to instruct on preventive exercises.

■ General Principles of Surgery

- Surgery often involves surgical extirpation of the primary tumor and removal of the regional lymphatics (neck dissection).
- Most common primary modality for oral cavity, thyroid, parotid, and sinonasal tumors with radiation and chemotherapy as adjuvant treatment.
- Important salvage modality for persistent disease of the larynx, oropharynx, hypopharynx, and cervical nodal disease.
- Neck dissection often considered in combination with chemoradiation for treatment of bulky N2–3 disease either planned or as salvage or elective treatment of early stage tumors especially of the oral cavity.

- Types of neck dissection include radical, modified radical, and selective.
- Microvascular reconstructive/oncoplastic surgery allows surgeons to be much more aggressive since large defects can now be reconstructed with form, function, and cosmesis.

■ General Principles of Medical Oncology

Chemotherapy is often incorporated in patients with stage III and IV cancers in patients treated with primary radiation therapy in one of the following scenarios:

- With radiation therapy (concurrent)
- Before radiation therapy (induction)
- Concurrent with radiation after surgery (adjuvant)
- As single-modality therapy for patients with locoregionally recurrent or metastatic disease

Chemotherapy:

- Improves survival and organ preservation in patients with locally advanced head and neck cancer.[1]
- Decreases distant failure.
- Most common agents include:
  - Cisplatin
  - Taxanes
  - 5-Fluorouracil
  - Methotrexate
  - Epidermal growth factor receptor inhibitors

■ General Principles of Radiation Therapy

- Radiation has electromagnetic properties similar to microwaves, radio waves, and light but it is distinguished by its ability to ionize and cause free radical formation, which results in breakup of tumor DNA.
- The most common radiation form is photons, which are generated by linear accelerators, which are high energy and able to spare skin and deliver the majority of the dose below the skin surface.

- Electrons are also used but deposit dose relatively more superficially and are commonly applied to skin cancers.
- Other forms of particle radiotherapy include protons, neutrons, and carbon ions, which will not apply in this textbook.
- Radiation that is implanted in head and neck tumors (brachytherapy) includes iridium 192 and iodine-125 isotopes, which deliver radiation over a small area of 3–5 millimeters.
- Radiation dose is measured in grays (Gy) or centigrays (cGy, 1/100 of Gy).
- Typical doses of radiation to treat head and neck cancer usually require 66–70 Gy (gross disease), 60–63 Gy (microscopic disease), and 50–54 Gy (elective treatment) depending on tumor burden.
- Fractionation refers to the schedule of radiation dosing.
- Conventional fractionation typically involves the delivery of 70 Gy in seven weeks over 35 treatments (Monday–Friday with weekends off).
- Altered fractionation either shortens overall treatment time (typically to six weeks) with the same total dose to minimize tumor repopulation or involves hyperfractionation, giving multiple daily fractions (typically 2 per day) to allow dose escalation (typically an extra 10 Gy) without increasing long-term side effects.
- Treatment breaks of more than five days detracts from the ability of radiation to control tumor and should be avoided.
- Intensity-modulated radiation therapy represents an important technique to deliver photon radiation to treat complex, irregularly shaped tumors such as in the oropharynx and nasopharynx while sparing normal tissue.
- It involves computed tomography guidance, delineation of tumor, areas at risk for tumor involvement, and normal tissues to be avoided.
- Radiation beams of various angles, intensities, and shapes are generated from treatment planning software to deliver high doses of radiation to the tumor and nodal

stations while sparing/limiting dose to normal tissues such as spinal cord, constrictor muscles, salivary glands, cochlea, visual pathways, and brain.

▪ Intensity modulated radiation therapy improves tumor control and reduces toxicity to swallowing, salivary flow, hearing, and mastication, which translates into improvement in quality of life.[2,3,4]

■ Toxicity

Medical Oncology

▪ Chemotherapy used to treat head and neck cancer carries significant risk, including:
  1. Nausea, vomiting, and diarrhea
  2. Bone marrow suppression, including anemia, neutropenia, and thrombocytopenia
  3. Mucositis
  4. Fatigue
  5. Organ dysfunction and failure, including that of the kidneys, liver, and lungs
  6. Skin toxicity (epidermal growth factor reception inhibitors)

▪ Smokers and heavy drinkers are at increased risk for emphysema, pneumonia, and liver failure.

▪ Performance status is a crucial predictor of tolerance to high-dose chemotherapy.

▪ Age is also important and there might be less benefit to chemotherapy after age 70 in head and neck cancer[5]even though the authors of this book do not routinely use age to determine suitability for chemotherapy.

Radiation Therapy

Acute
  1. Mucositis/pain/odynophagia
  2. Phlegm production, which can trigger coughing/nausea/vomiting
  3. Dysgeusia and xerostomia
  4. Weight loss/dehydration
  5. Fatigue
  6. Dermatitis

Chronic

1. Xerostomia
2. Swallowing dysfunction
3. Strictures, feeding tube dependence
4. Dental caries/osteoradionecrosis
5. Neck fibrosis/trismus
6. Hypothyroidism
7. Epilation

■ Follow-up

▣ Greatest risk of recurrence is during the first 2 years after treatment.

▣ Secondary malignancies at a rate of 7–15% especially if smoking continues.

▣ Follow-up visits:
  - Every 1–2 months first year
  - Every 2–3 months second year, every 3–6 months years 3–5, then annually
  - Thyrotropin (TSH) q 6 months first 2 years then yearly afterward
  - Baseline cross-sectional imaging posttreatment, yearly chest x-ray and additional studies as indicated
  - Dental prophylaxis and speech/swallowing evaluation as needed

■ References

1. Haddad RI, Shin DM. Recent advances in head and neck cancer. *N Engl J Med.* 2008;359(11):1143–1154.
2. Eisbruch A, Kim HM, Terrell JE. Xerostomia and its predictors following parotid-sparing irradiation of head-and-neck cancer. *Int J Radiat Oncol Biol Phys.* 2001;50(3):695–704.
3. Chen WC, Jackson A, Budnick AS. Sensorineural hearing loss in combined modality treatment of nasopharyngeal carcinoma. *Cancer.* 2006;106(4):820–829.
4. Feng FY, Kim HM, Lyden TH, et al. Intensity-modulated chemoradiotherapy aiming to reduce dysphagia in patients with oropharyngeal cancer: clinical and functional results. *J Clin Oncol.* 2010;28(16):2732–2738.
5. Pignon JP, le Maitre A, Bourhis J. Meta-analyses of chemotherapy in head and neck cancer (MACH-NC): an update. *Int J Radiat Oncol Biol Phys.* 2007;69(2 Suppl):S112–S114.

Management of the Neck

■ Introduction

- Elective or therapeutic treatment of the neck is usually required for the cure of most head and neck squamous cell carcinomas.
- Elective treatment with either radiotherapy or surgery is required in clinically negative necks because of the high risk for occult cervical nodal spread.
- Therapeutic treatment involves multimodality therapy—typically a combination of surgery, radiotherapy, and chemotherapy.
- Management of the neck follows the manner in which the primary tumors treated.
- Nodal involvement decreases the risk of cure by one half.[1]

■ Nodal Staging and Nodal Stations at Risk

- American Joint Cancer Committee neck staging system emphasizes the importance of node size, multiplicity of nodes, and spread to the contralateral neck (**Table 2.1**).
- The international consensus nodal station levels are illustrated in **Figure 2.1**.
- Nodal level stations as outlined by radiographically identifiable landmarks (see **Figure 2.2**).
- Incidence of nodal involvement of the most common head and neck cancer sites (see **Table 2.2**).[2]
- In clinically negative necks:
  - Levels II and III are at greatest risk for occult nodal disease for larynx cancers.

Table 2.1 **AJCC 2010 Neck Staging for Nonnasopharynx Cancer Sites**

Stage	Nodal Involvement
N0	No involved node
N1	Single ipsilateral node ≤ 3 cm
N2	a. Single ipsilateral node > 3 cm, ≤ 6 cm b. Multiple ipsilateral nodes all ≤ 6 cm c. Bilateral or contralateral nodes ≤ 6 cm
N3	Node > 6 cm

Source: Edge SB, Byrd DR, Compton CC, eds. *AJCC Cancer Staging Handbook.* 7th ed. New York, NY: Springer, 2010, Chapter 5, page 70.

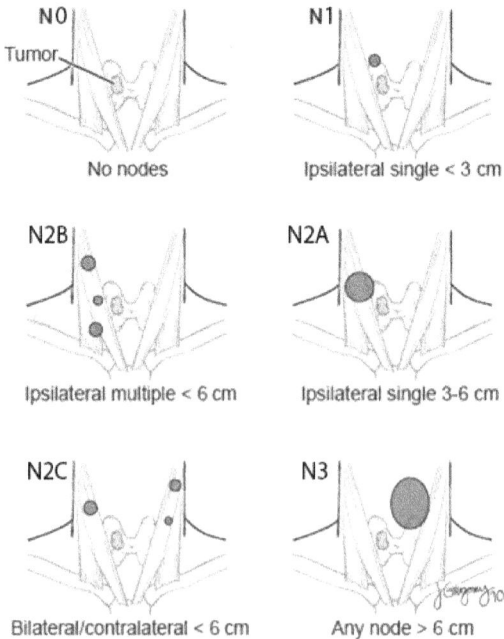

Figure 2.1 Neck Nodal Level Classification
Nodal drainage levels as determined by radiographically based landmarks.
Source: Courtesy of Jill K. Gregory, Continuum Health Partners.

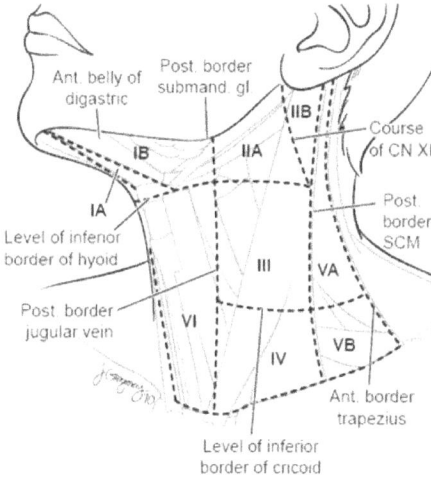

Figure 2.2 AJCC Neck Nodal Staging
Source: Courtesy of Jill K. Gregory, Continuum Health Partners.

Table 2.2   Percentage Incidence and Distribution of Pathologically Involved Nodes in a Clinical Node Negative Neck after Elective Radical Neck Dissection

	I	II	III	IV	V
Oropharynx n = 48	2	25	19	8	2
Hypopharynx n = 24	0	13	13	0	0
Larynx n = 79	5	19	20	9	2.5
Oral Cavity n = 192	20	17	9	3	0.5

Source: Shah JP et al. The patterns of cervical lymph node metastases from squamous carcinoma of the oral cavity. *Cancer.* 1990;66(1):109–113.

- Levels II–IV are at greatest risk for oropharynx and hypopharynx cancers.
- Levels I–III are at greatest risk for oral cavity cancers.
▪ In clinically node-positive patients:
  - The risk for level IV nodal involvement increases in larynx and oral cavity cancer patients.

Table 2.3 **Percentage Incidence and Distribution of Pathologically Involved Nodes in a Clinical Node Positive after Therapeutic Radical Neck Dissection**

	I	II	III	IV	V
Oropharynx n = 165	14	71	42	28	9
Larynx n = 183	7	57	59	29	4
Hypopharynx n = 104	10	76	73	46	11
Oral Cavity n = 324	46	43	33	15	3

Source: Shah JP. Patterns of cervical lymph node metastasis from squamous carcinomas of the upper aerodigestive tract. *Am J Surg*. 1990;160(4):405–409.

- Levels I and V become increasingly involved in oropharynx and hypopharynx (**Table 2.3**).
- In general, patients with clinically node-positive disease require bilateral neck management.
- Unilateral neck treatment is usually reserved for well-lateralized lesions such as small oral cavity or oropharynx lesions and parotid cancers.

Elective Treatment of the Clinically Node-Negative Neck

- Both selective neck dissection and elective nodal irradiation (ENI) represent excellent options to address clinically occult regional disease.[3,4]
- Surgery offers important pathologic data that is useful prognostically and tailors further therapy according to risk stratification.
- Radiation adds more comprehensive nodal coverage including the contralateral neck and in regions difficult to surgically address such as the retropharyngeal nodes.

Surgical Details of Elective Neck Dissection

▨ There are three different types of neck dissections.
1. *Radical neck dissection.* Removes levels I–V nodes in continuity with the sternocleidomastoid muscle, spinal accessory nerve, and internal jugular vein.
2. *Modified radical neck dissections.* Removes levels I–V nodes but spares the following:
   ▨ Spinal accessory nerve (type I)
   ▨ Spinal accessory and internal jugular vein (type II)
   ▨ Spinal accessory, internal jugular vein, and sternocleidomastoid muscle (type III)
3. *Selective neck dissection (SND).* Removes only nodal levels at highest risk for occult disease and preserves spinal accessory nerve, sternocleidomastoid muscle, and internal jugular vein.

Radiation Therapy Details of Elective Nodal Radiation

▨ ENI usually entails treatment to a dose of 50 Gy to nodal stations determined by the primary site.[4,5]
▨ Bilateral ENI is used for larynx (except early stage glottis larynx) and hypopharynx cancers and should be considered for tumors arising from the soft palate, base of tongue, and pharyngeal wall which often extend up to and past midline.
▨ In ipsilateral cancers, ENI is warranted for small lateralized oral cavity and oropharynx disease with N0–1 necks.[6,7]
▨ The efficacy of ENI shows no obvious differences compared to elective neck dissection.[8]

■ Definitive Management of the Clinically Node-Positive Neck

Management Options

▨ Management of the clinical positive neck involves multiple options, including:
   • Neck dissection followed by postoperative radiation with or without chemotherapy
   • Definitive radiation or concurrent chemoradiation with close surveillance with positron emission

tomography/computed tomography. Neck dissection may be incorporated as a planned approach or salvage of residual disease. It is highly recommended in these situations that the PET scan is obtained at a minimum of 12 weeks post chemoradiotherapy to decrease the high false positive and negative rates that occur if the PET scan is done before that. Surgical experience in the management of a radiated neck is important.

- Factors that determine how best to manage the neck include the resectability of the primary and neck disease, the functional morbidity incurred by surgery or radiation at the primary site, and the appropriateness of the primary lesion for potential organ-preserving therapy with either radiation alone or in combination with chemotherapy.
- When unresectable disease exists, the use of sequential or concurrent chemoradiotherapy is largely favored.

Surgical Details of Therapeutic Neck Dissection

- The type of therapeutic neck dissection depends on the nodal burden and levels of involvement.
- If there is a heavy volume of disease within the lymph nodes on imaging, a comprehensive neck dissection is performed (radical neck dissection vs modified radical neck dissection).
- If the internal jugular vein or the sternocleidomastoid muscle appears involved on preoperative imaging, they are usually sacrificed during the surgery in an attempt to perform an en bloc resection.
- Attempts to preserve the spinal accessory nerve are considered if the nerve is not involved by tumor.

The Role of Radiation Therapy

Radiation therapy may be used as adjuvant or for the definitive management of the node-positive neck.

Surgery and Postoperative Radiation

- Surgery and postoperative radiation remain a common strategy for regional management, especially for the majority of resectable oral cavity tumors, bulky or cartilage invasive hypopharynx, and larynx cancers.

* Risk factors for recurrence include positive margins, extracapsular extension of nodal disease, multiple nodes, lymph-vascular or perineural invasion, T3–4 primary lesion, time interval more than six weeks between surgery and beginning of radiation therapy.[8,9]

* Extracapsular extension and/or positive margins are the greatest risk factors for recurrence and require intensification of treatment with shortened total treatment package times,[10] radiation dose escalation,[11] or concurrent chemoradiation.[12–14]

Postop Chemoradiation for High-Risk Disease

* Two landmark clinical trials have demonstrated that in patients with high-risk disease, the addition of three cycles of high-dose cisplatin concurrent with postoperative radiation increases locoregional control, disease-free survival, and overall survival compared to post-operative radiation alone (**Table 2.4**).[12,13]

* The addition of cisplatin increases the incidence of severe mucositis and acute symptoms with a small but significant risk for treatment-related mortality.

* Long-term side effects were no different.

* In a pooled analysis of the two studies,[14] extracapsular extension of tumor and positive margins were the only factors in which clear-cut benefit could be achieved with the addition of cisplatin.

* Standard chemotherapy consists of 3 cycles of high-dose cisplatin at 100 mg/m^2 given on days 1, 22, and 43 of postoperative radiation therapy to a dose of 60–66 Gy over seven weeks.

■ Primary Radiation Treatment of the Node-Positive Neck

Radiation Therapy with or without Chemotherapy

* For N1 patients, definitive radiation offers disease control in 90% and does not appear to differ compared to those undergoing neck dissection.[15]

Table 2.4 Comparison of Phase III Postoperative Chemoradiation vs Radiation

	RTOG 95-01	EORTC 22931
Number of patients	459	334
Pt characteristic		
OPX/OC/LX/HPX	42%/27%/21%/10%	30%/26%/22%/20%
% T3–4	61%	66%
% N2–3	94%	57%
High-Risk Criteria		
% with ECE – margin	49%	41%
% with + margins – ECE	6%	13%
% with ECE and + margins	4%	16%
% with ECE and/or + margins	59%	70%
RT: % receiving 66 Gy	13%	91%
≥ grade 3 acute toxicity (CT/RT vs RT)	77% vs 34% (p < 0.0001)	44% vs 21% (p = 0.001)
All late toxicity (CT/RT vs RT)	21% vs 17% (p = 0.29)	38% vs 41% (p = 0.25)
Median follow-up	46 mo	60 mo
Outcomes (CT/RT vs RT)		
Locoregional failure	3 yr: 22% vs 33% (p = 0.01)	5 yr: 18% vs 31% (p = 0.007)
Disease-free survival	3 yr: 47% vs 36% (p = 0.04)	5 yr: 47% vs 36% (p = 0.04)

Table 2.4   Comparison of Phase III Postoperative Chemoradiation vs Radiation (Continued)

	RTOG 95-01	EORTC 22931
Overall survival	3 yr: 56% vs 47% (p = 0.09)	5 yr: 53% vs 40% (p = 0.02)
Distant metastases	3 yr: 20% vs 23% (p = 0.46)	5 yr: 21% vs 24% (p = 0.61)

OPX = oropharynx; OC = oral cavity; LX = larynx; HPX = hypopharynx; ECE = extracapsular extension; p = p value; CT = chemotherapy; RT = radiation therapy.

Source: Cooper JS, Pajak TF, Forastiere AA, et al. Postoperative concurrent radiotherapy and chemotherapy for high-risk squamous-cell carcinoma of the head and neck. *N Engl J Med.* 2004;350:1934–1937; Bernier J, Domenge C, Ozsahin M, et al. Postoperative irradiation with or without concomitant chemotherapy for locally advanced head and neck cancer. *N Engl J Med.* 2004;350:1945–1952.

- For N2–3 patients, chemoradiation is often considered especially if the primary site is treated similarly.
- Confirmation of a complete nodal response with positron emission tomography/computed tomography at 3 months after treatment is crucial to ensure excellent regional control.
- A neck dissection following radiation therapy may be considered in those with bulky N2 or N3 disease either as a planned approach or as salvage for incomplete response.
- The primary complications that may occur from definitive neck radiation treatment include fibrosis, brachial plexopathy and increased wound complications if neck dissection is required for persistent disease.

Role of Intensity-Modulated Radiation Therapy in the Management of the Neck

- The greatest advantage to using intensity-modulated radiation therapy in managing the neck is to spare parotid glands in the node-negative neck by omitting the high jugular nodes which are adjacent to the parotid.

- Consensus guidelines have been reached to spare the high jugular nodes in a node-negative neck and are illustrated in Figure 2.1.
- Recently, the identification of dose constraints to the constrictor muscles have made swallowing function preservation a potential benefit in intensity-modulated radiation therapy–treated patients.

■ Management of Recurrent Neck Disease

- Recurrent squamous cell carcinoma in the neck is difficult to salvage for multiple reasons, including the high risk for concurrent distant metastases or local failure, unresectability of the regional site due to carotid artery encasement, and treatment resistance due to prior multimodality therapy.
- Surgical salvage is worthwhile especially if it can be combined with radiation and/or chemotherapy.
- To minimize wound complications and to allow better tolerance to adjuvant therapy, incorporation of flap reconstruction techniques is recommended.[16,17]
- Typical reconstruction methods include pedicle myocutaneous flaps[18] or microvascular-free flaps,[19] which optimize wound healing with improved vascularization from unirradiated tissue.[20,21]
- If patients have been previously irradiated with external beam, reirradiation with brachytherapy (placement of radioactive sources directly into the tumor bed) can improve neck control with low morbidity.
- Brachytherapy may involve temporary placement of radiation catheters through which iridium 192 sources are placed, permanent seed implantation with iodine 125 sutures or intraoperative radiation therapy techniques.
- Distant metastasis and locoregional failure outside of the treatment area remain significant.
- Chemotherapy is usually recommended in conjunction with external-beam radiation therapy if patients are eligible.

■ References

1. Cachin Y, Sancho-Garnier H, Micheau C, et al. Nodal metastasis from carcinomas of the oropharynx. *Otolaryngol Clin North Am.* 1979;12(1):145–154.
2. Shah, JP. Patterns of cervical lymph node metastasis from squamous carcinomas of the upper aerodigestive tract. *Am J Surg.* 1990;160(4):405–409.
3. Byers RM. Modified neck dissection. A study of 967 cases from 1970 to 1980. *Am J Surg.* 1985;150(4):414–421.
4. Fletcher GH. Elective irradiation of subclinical disease in cancers of the head and neck. *Cancer.* 1972;29(6):1450–1454.
5. Mendenhall WM, Million RR, Cassisi, NJ. Elective neck irradiation in squamous-cell carcinoma of the head and neck. *Head Neck Surg.* 1980;3(1):15–20.
6. O'Sullivan B, Warde P, Grice B, et al. The benefits and pitfalls of ipsilateral radiotherapy in carcinoma of the tonsillar region. *Int J Radiat Oncol Biol Phys.* 2001;51(2):332–343.
7. Armstrong JG, Harrison LB, Thaler HT, et al. The indications for elective treatment of the neck in cancer of the major salivary glands. *Cancer.* 1992;69(3):615–619.
8. Barkley HT Jr, Fletcher GH, Jesse RH, et al. Management of cervical lymph node metastases in squamous cell carcinoma of the tonsillar fossa, base of tongue, supraglottic larynx, and hypopharynx. *Am J Surg.* 1972;124(4):462–467.
9. Vikram B, Strong EW, Shah JP, et al. Failure in the neck following multimodality treatment for advanced head and neck cancer. *Head Neck Surg.* 1984;6(3):724–729.
10. Ang KK, Trotti A, Brown BW, et al. Randomized trial addressing risk features and time factors of surgery plus radiotherapy in advanced head-and-neck cancer. *Int J Radiat Oncol Biol Phys.* 2001;51(3):571–578.
11. Peters LJ, Goepfert H, Ang KK, et al. Evaluation of the dose for postoperative radiation therapy of head and neck cancer: first report of a prospective randomized trial. *Int J Radiat Oncol Biol Phys.* 1993;26(1):3–11.
12. Cooper JS, Pajak TF, Forastiere AA, et al. Postoperative concurrent radiotherapy and chemotherapy for high-risk squamous-cell carcinoma of the head and neck. *N Engl J Med.* 2004;350(19):1937–1944.
13. Bernier J, Domenge C, Ozsahin M, et al. Postoperative irradiation with or without concomitant chemotherapy for locally advanced head and neck cancer. *N Engl J Med.* 2004;350(19):1945–1952.
14. Bernier J, Cooper JS, Pajak TF, et al. Defining risk levels in locally advanced head and neck cancers: a comparative analysis of concurrent postoperative radiation plus chemotherapy trials

of the EORTC (#22931) and RTOG (# 9501). *Head Neck.* 2005;27(10):843–850.

15. Mendenhall WM, Million RR, Cassisi NJ. Squamous cell carcinoma of the head and neck treated with radiation therapy: the role of neck dissection for clinically positive neck nodes. *Int J Radiat Oncol Biol Phys.* 1986;12(5):733–740.

16. Peters LJ, Weber RS, Morrison WH, et al. Neck surgery in patients with primary oropharyngeal cancer treated by radiotherapy. *Head Neck.* 1996;18(6):552–559.

17. Mendenhall WM, Million RR, Bova FJ. Analysis of time-dose factors in clinically positive neck nodes treated with irradiation alone in squamous cell carcinoma of the head and neck. *Int J Radiat Oncol Biol Phys.* 1984;10(5):639–643.

18. Stafford N, Dearnaley D. Treatment of 'inoperable' neck nodes using surgical clearance and postoperative interstitial irradiation. *Br J Surg.* 1988;75(1):62–64.

19. Moscoso JF, Urken ML, Dalton J, et al. Simultaneous interstitial radiotherapy with regional or free-flap reconstruction, following salvage surgery of recurrent head and neck carcinoma: analysis of complications. *Arch Otolaryngol Head Neck Surg.* 1994;120(9):965–972.

20. Vikram B, Strong EW, Shah JP, et al. Intraoperative radiotherapy in patients with recurrent head and neck cancer. *Am J Surg.* 1985;150(4):485–487.

21. Chen KY, Mohr RM, Silverman CL. Interstitial iodine 125 in advanced recurrent squamous cell carcinoma of the head and neck with follow-up evaluation of carotid artery by ultrasound. *Ann Otol Rhinol Laryngol.* 1996;105(12):955–961.

22. Harrison LB, Sessions RB, Hong WK. *Head and Neck Cancer: A Multidisciplinary Approach.* Lippincott Williams & Wilkins; 2008, Boston, MA.

Oral Cavity Cancer

▣ Anatomy

- ▣ Although the oral cavity is relatively small in size, it is anatomically a challenging region because of the wide range of tissues and functions of its structures.
- ▣ It begins at the vermilion border of the lips and extends posteriorly to the junction of the hard and soft palate.
- ▣ It consists of the following:
  - The lips
  - The oral tongue (anterior to circumvallate papilla)
  - The floor of the mouth
  - The buccal mucosa
  - The retromolar trigone
  - The hard palate
  - The gingiva

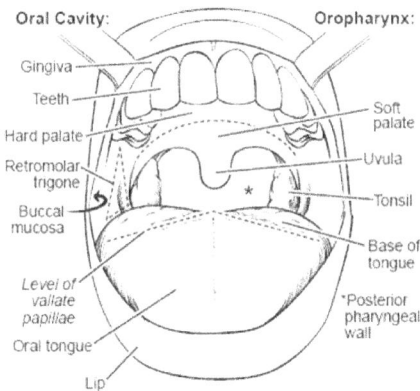

Figure 3.1 Anatomy of Oral Cavity
Subsites comprising the oral cavity are delineated. The circumvallate papillae mark the border between the oropharyngeal base of the tongue and the oral tongue.
Source: Courtesy of Jill K. Gregory, Continuum Health Partners.

- Cancer and the treatment of a cancer within the oral cavity can have a tremendous impact on a patient's ability to maintain nutrition, communicate, and interact socially with other people.
- Therefore, the impact of the various treatment options for a cancer of the oral cavity must take into consideration the potential impact on the patient's quality of life and function preservation.

Incidence and Risk Factors

- Squamous cell carcinoma, which originates from the mucosal lining of the oral cavity, remains by far the most common type of carcinoma of the oral cavity, accounting for over 95%.
- The next most common origin is from the minor salivary glands, which are dispersed throughout the oral cavity.
- Tobacco and alcohol are the major risk factors.
- Although it is not common practice in the United States, betel nut chewing is also strongly associated with cancer of the oral cavity.
- Leukoplakia and erythroplakia are premalignant conditions that warrant close observation with malignant progression in 4–18% and 30%, respectively.

Signs and Symptoms

- The most common presentation of an oral cavity cancer is a nonhealing ulcer.
- As the lesion progresses, the patient often develops tongue pain, dysarthria, odynophagia, ear pain, weight loss, and appetite loss.

Staging

Primary Tumor (T)

- TX: Primary tumor cannot be assessed.
- T0: No evidence of primary tumor.
- Tis: Carcinoma in situ.
- T1: Tumor 2 cm or less in greatest dimension.

- T2: Tumor more than 2 cm but not more than 4 cm in greatest dimension.
- T3: Tumor more than 4 cm in greatest dimension.
- T4: Lip tumor invades adjacent structures (e.g., through cortical bone, inferior alveolar nerve, the floor of the mouth, the skin of the face). Oral cavity tumor invades adjacent structures (e.g., through cortical bone, into deep muscles of the tongue, maxillary sinus, or skin).

Regional Lymph Nodes (N)

- NX: Regional lymph nodes cannot be assessed.
- N0: No regional lymph node metastasis.
- N1: Metastasis in a single ipsilateral lymph node, 3 cm or less in greatest dimension.
- N2: Metastasis in a single ipsilateral lymph node, more than 3 cm but not more than 6 cm in greatest dimension; or in multiple ipsilateral lymph nodes, none more than 6 cm in greatest dimension; or in bilateral or contralateral lymph nodes, none more than 6 cm in greatest dimension.
  - N2a: Metastasis in a single ipsilateral lymph node more than 3 cm but not more than 6 cm in dimension
  - N2b: Metastasis in multiple ipsilateral lymph nodes, none more than 6 cm in greatest dimension.
  - N2c: Metastasis in bilateral or contralateral lymph nodes, none more than 6 cm in greatest dimension
  - N3: Metastasis in a lymph node more than 6 cm in greatest dimension

Distant Metastasis (M)

- MX: Presence of distant metastasis cannot be assessed
- M0: No distant metastasis
- M1: Distant metastasis

Stage

Stage I:	T1	N0	M0
Stage II:	T2	N0	M0
Stage III:	T3	N1	M0
Stage IV:	T4	N2	M1

■ Treatment

- Oral cavity cancers are generally approached surgically as the primary modality of therapy.
- Early cancers (stage I and II) can often be treated with unimodal therapy; i.e., surgery alone.
- Advanced cancers (stage III and IV) generally require multimodality therapy; i.e., surgery followed by radiation with or without chemotherapy.

Surgery

- Tumors in the oral cavity are generally easy to access transorally if they are small in size.
- As the tumors become larger and involve more of the structures of the oral cavity, an open approach to the oral cavity with mandibulotomy or mandibular resection is required.
- Additionally, when cancers of the oral cavity are treated, they generally require external incision for a cervical lymphadenectomy.
- Each subsite of the oral cavity can be approached in a variety of ways.

Tongue

1. Partial glossectomy with primary closure
2. Partial glossectomy with split-thickness skin graft reconstruction
3. Partial glossectomy requiring the transfer of tissue (radial forearm free flap) to reconstitute volume loss and prevent tethering of the tongue to the floor of the mouth
4. Total glossectomy requiring tissue transfer to create a neotongue

Mandible

1. Marginal mandibulectomy
2. Segmental mandibulectomy
3. Composite resection of tongue/floor of mouth with a segment of mandible

Lip

1. Wedge resection with primary closure
2. Wide resection requiring lip reconstruction

Floor of Mouth

1. Wide resection with primary closure
2. Wide resection with split-thickness skin graft reconstruction
3. Wide resection requiring the transfer of tissue to prevent tethering of the tongue
4. Composite resection of tongue/floor of mouth/mandible requiring a complex reconstruction with tissue transfer

Hard Palate

1. Wide resection of lining of hard palate
2. Wide resection of lining of hard palate requiring underlying bone to be resected
3. Infrastructure maxillectomy requiring obturation or reconstruction with a free tissue transfer

■ Goals of Reconstruction

- *Mandible*: Reconstitution of the mandibular arch to preserve form and function. To provide a platform for implant-borne or a tissue-borne prosthesis to be created for dental rehabilitation
- *Tongue*: To create a neotongue with enough volume and mobility to adequately oppose the palate and manipulate a food bolus
- *Hard palate*: To patch or obturate a connection created between the sinonasal cavity and the oral cavity
- *Floor of mouth*: To minimize tethering of the tongue
- *Lip*: To maintain oral competence

■ Postoperative Adjuvant Therapy

Intermediate Risk Factors

- Adverse pathologic factors such perineural/lymph-vascular invasion, T3–4, margins < 5 mm and multiple nodes are deemed intermediate risk and require adjuvant radiation therapy.[1]
- Radiation therapy addresses the primary site and neck(s) as appropriate to doses ranging from 60 to 66 Gy over six to seven weeks.

High Risk

- Extracapsular extension of nodal disease and positive margins are deemed high risk and warrant concurrent chemoradiation.[2,3]
- Some patients will fall into a gray area of intermediate or high risk.
- Patients who are poor candidates for standard chemoradiation may be treated with weekly doses of platinum-based drugs.
- In a total treatment package, timing of surgery to the end of radiation therapy should ideally be kept to 11 weeks or less in high-risk patients to optimize locoregional control and survival requiring patients to start treatment within 4 weeks of surgery.
- Chemoradiation consists of high-dose cisplatin 100 mg/m^2 q three weeks for three cycles on days 1, 22, and 43 of a seven-week course of radiation to doses of 60–66 Gy.
- Two landmark trials (EORT 22931 and RTOG 95-01) demonstrated a locoregional control and survival benefit of the regimen for high-risk head and neck squamous cell carcinomas including oral cavity cancers (**Figure 3.2** and **Table 3.1**).[2,3]

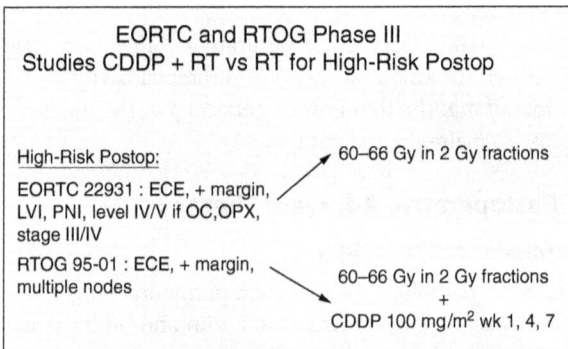

EORTC and RTOG Phase III
Studies CDDP + RT vs RT for High-Risk Postop

High-Risk Postop:

EORTC 22931 : ECE, + margin, LVI, PNI, level IV/V if OC,OPX, stage III/IV → 60–66 Gy in 2 Gy fractions

RTOG 95-01 : ECE, + margin, multiple nodes → 60–66 Gy in 2 Gy fractions + CDDP 100 mg/m^2 wk 1, 4, 7

Figure 3.2 Definition of Pathologic Factors for High Risk of Failure
Both cooperative groups defined ECE and positive margins as high risk. CDDP = cisplatin; RT = external beam radiation; ECE = extracapsular invasion; LVI = lymph-vascular invasion; PNI = perineural invasion; OC = oral cavity; OPX = oropharynx.

Table 3.1   Postop CT/RT vs RT: Results of EORTC/RTOG Phase III Trials

	RTOG 95-01	EORTC 22931
Median Followup	46 mo	60 mo
Locoregional Failure	Outcomes (CT/RT vs RT) 3 yr : 22% vs 33% (p = 0.01)	Outcomes (CT/RT vs RT) 5 yr :18% vs 31% (p = 0.007)
Disease-Free Survival	3 yr :47% vs 36% (p = 0.04)	5 yr :47% vs 36% (p = 0.04)
Overall Survival	3 yr :56% vs 47% (p = 0.09)	5 yr :53% vs 40% (p = 0.02)
Distant Metastases	3 yr :20% vs 23% (p = 0.46)	5 yr :21% vs 24% (p = 0.61)
≥ Grade 3 Acute Toxicity	77% vs 34% (p < 0.0001)	44% vs 21% (p = 0.001)
All Late Toxicity	21% vs 17% (p = 0.29)	38% vs 41% (p = 0.25)

Comparison of outcomes from the RTOG 95-01 and EORTC 22931. Both groups showed the addition of concurrent chemotherapy improved locoregional control and disease-free survival.

Source: Cooper JS, Pajak TF, Forastiere AA, et al. Postoperative concurrent radiotherapy and chemotherapy for high-risk squamous-cell carcinoma of the head and neck. *N Engl J Med*. 2004;350:1937–1934; Bernier J, Domenge C, Ozsahin M, et al. Postoperative irradiation with or without concomitant chemotherapy for locally advanced head and neck cancer. *N Engl J Med*. 2004;350:1945–1952.

- Acute grade 3 or greater toxicities were doubled in the chemoradiation arm and consisted primarily of mucositis, hematologic toxicity, nephropathy, and ototoxicity.
- No difference in late toxicity was reported.
- There is about a 2% incidence of treatment-related mortality in patients undergoing chemoradiation highlighting the importance of multidisciplinary supportive care as well as the need for an adequate baseline performance status.

■ Definitive Radiation Therapy

■ Primary radiation therapy is an alternative treatment for patients who refuse or are not surgical candidates.

■ In such setting, the best outcomes have incorporated brachytherapy implant into the primary site combined with external beam radiation or neck dissection to address regional disease.

■ For advanced primary lesions or those with nodal disease, a course of external beam radiation with or without chemotherapy or biologic therapy.

■ Incorporation of brachytherapy after external beam treatment of oral cavity cancers allows higher doses of radiation to be delivered (often 77–80 Gy) than can be achieved with external beam radiation.

■ In select situations, brachytherapy alone combined with a selective neck dissection can be used to treat oral cavity cancers, especially if the tumors are small and there are no clinically involved nodes (**Figure 3.3**).

■ Outcomes from large brachytherapy series involving treatment of the lip, oral tongue, and floor of mouth show similar outcomes to surgically treated patients.[4–6]

■ However, the brachytherapy technique requires special expertise and should be done with an experienced radiation oncologist.

■ References

1. Ang KK, Trotti A, Brown BW, et al. Randomized trial addressing risk features and time factors of surgery plus radiotherapy in advanced head-and-neck cancer. *Int J Radiat Oncol Biol Phys.* 2001;51:571–578.

2. Cooper JS, Pajak TF, Forastiere AA, et al. Postoperative concurrent radiotherapy and chemotherapy for high-risk squamous-cell carcinoma of the head and neck. *N Engl J Med.* 2004;350:1937–1934.

3. Bernier J, Domenge C, Ozsahin M, et al. Postoperative irradiation with or without concomitant chemotherapy for locally advanced head and neck cancer. *N Engl J Med.* 2004;350:1945–1952.

4. Decroix Y, Ghossein NA. Experience of the Curie Institute in treatment of cancer of the mobile tongue: I. Treatment policies and result. *Cancer.* 1981;47(3):496–502.

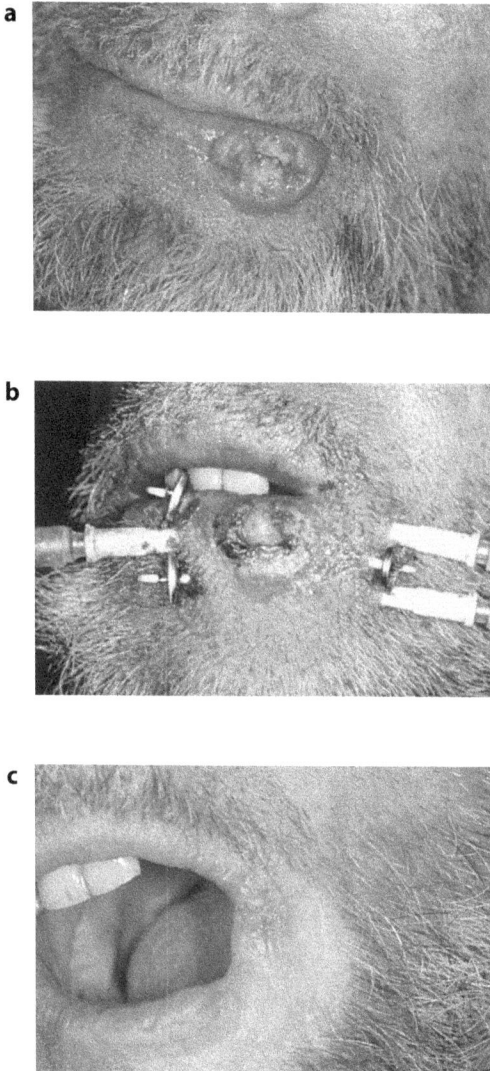

Figure 3.3 Brachytherapy Treatment Alone for a Lip Squamous Cell Carcinoma

(a) T1 cancer involving the lower lip near the oral commissure without nodal disease on imaging. (b) An interstitial implant with three catheters in which Ir-192 ribbons are loaded. A total dose of 60 Gy was delivered. (c) One month postbrachytherapy showing complete response of the tumor with healing mucositis.

5. Pernot M, Hoffstetter S, Peiffert D, et al. Epidermoid carcinomas of the floor of mouth treated by exclusive irradiation: statistical study of a series of 207 cases. *Radiother Oncol.* 1995;35(3):177–185.
6. Jorgensen K, Elbronad O, Anderson AP. Carcinoma of the lip: a series of 869 cases. *Acta Radiol Ther Phys Biol.* 1973;12:177–190.

Oropharynx

■ Introduction

▩ Cancers of the oropharynx are common.

▩ The oropharynx is comprised of four different sites, including the soft palate, the tonsillar region (fossa and pillars), the base of the tongue, and the posterior and lateral pharyngeal wall between the nasopharynx and the larynx (see **Figure 4.1**).

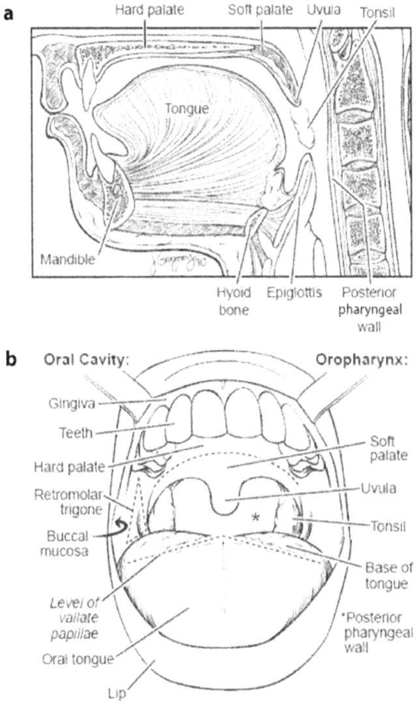

Figure 4.1 Anatomy of Oropharynx Cancer
(a) Lateral view of the oropharynx, showing the posterior pharyngeal wall.
(b) Anterior view of the oropharynx.
Source: Courtesy of Jill K. Gregory, Continuum Health Partners.

- Of these, the two sites that are most commonly involved are the base of the tongue and the tonsils.
- Smoking and alcohol abuse are the major risk factors in developing oropharynx cancer.
- Recently, infection with the human papillomavirus (HPV), especially HPV-16, has been recognized as the predominant risk factor for oropharynx in the Western world.[1,2]
- It is currently estimated that in 50–60% of patients with oropharynx cancer, the cancer is HPV related.
- The major characteristics of HPV related oropharynx cancer are[3]:
  - Patients are about 10 years younger than those with a smoking/alcohol-related oropharynx cancer.
  - Patients are often nontobacco smokers and nondrinkers.
  - Pathology specimen often has a basaloid appearance.
  - Prognosis is excellent; cure rates often exceed 85% in patients whose disease is HPV related despite locally advanced disease.[4,5]
  - The excellent prognosis has led to the development of clinical trials targeted specifically toward patients with HPV.
  - Until those trials are completed, treatment should not be modified based on HPV status.
- The HPV status can be checked via fluorescent in situ hybridization or polymerase chain reaction techniques.
- Alternatively, p16 immunohistochemistry can serve as a surrogate for HPV infection and can be used to assess HPV status.[6]
- These tests are all performed on the surgical specimen.
- It is strongly recommended that the HPV status of all patients with oropharynx cancer is checked given its prognostic implications.

■ Signs and Symptoms

- Sore throat, dysphagia, and odynophagia and ear pain
- Painless neck node
- Trismus

■ Staging

American Joint Committee on Cancer tumor, node, metastasis classification of carcinoma of the oropharynx

- Primary tumor cannot be accessed.
- No evidence of primary tumor.
- Tis carcinoma in situ.
- T1: Tumor ≤ 2 cm in greatest dimension.
- T2: Tumor > 2 cm but ≤ 4 cm in greatest dimension.
- T3: Tumor > 4 cm in greatest dimension.
- T4a: Tumor involves masticator space, pterygoid plates, or skull base, and/or encases internal carotid artery.
- T4b: Tumor involves lateral pterygoid muscle, pterygoid plates, lateral nasopharynx, skull base, and/or encases internal carotid artery.
- Nx: Regional lymph nodes cannot be assessed.
- N0: No regional lymph node metastasis.
- N1: Metastasis in a single ipsilateral lymph node; ≤ 3 cm in greatest dimension.
- N2a: Metastasis in a single ipsilateral lymph node; > 3 cm but ≤ 6 cm in greatest dimension.
- NN2b: Metastasis in multiple ipsilateral lymph nodes; none > 6 cm in greatest dimension.
- N2c: Metastasis in bilateral or contralateral lymph nodes; none > 6 cm in greatest dimension.
- N3: Metastasis in a lymph node; > 6 cm in greatest dimension.
- M0: No distant metastasis.
- M1: Distant metastasis.

■ Treatment of Early Stage Disease: Stage I and II

- Either radiation therapy or surgical resection.
- Chemotherapy is rarely used in treating early stage oropharynx cancer.
- Cure rate often exceeds 90%.

External-Beam Radiation Therapy

- Primary radiation therapy is a standard approach as it addresses the large areas of potential nodal and local tumor spread while preserving organ function and integrity.

- For example, bilateral cervical and retropharyngeal nodes are commonly involved while tumors of the tonsil can spread to the insertion sites of the tonsil muscles at the skull base.[7]
- For early stage patients, radiation therapy alone to a dose of 66–70 Gy controls 80–90% of T1 and T2 lesions.[8–11]
- Lateralized small tonsil lesions with an N0 or N1 neck are treated with ipsilateral radiation fields.[12]
- A unilateral approach minimizes irradiation to the contralateral salivary glands and reduces the incidence of xerostomia.[13]
- Lesions that cross the midline, extensively involve the tongue base or soft palate, or associated with N2 or more advanced neck disease should receive comprehensive bilateral neck therapy.
- Patients with early stage tongue base, posterior pharyngeal, or soft palate lesions usually require bilateral treatment.
- In cases requiring bilateral neck radiation, intensity-modulated radiation therapy is the preferred treatment technique to spare the salivary glands and constrictor muscles important for swallowing while achieving rates of locoregional control over 90%.[12-17]

Brachytherapy for Oropharynx Cancer

- Brachytherapy is the direct implantation of radioactive seeds into the tumor.
- Brachytherapy allows dose escalation to the tumor and spares normal tissue by minimizing dose to surrounding normal tissue and lowering the total external-beam radiation needed to treat the tumor.
- With a combined brachytherapy and external-beam radiation therapy approach, typically 77–80 Gy are delivered to the primary site while 54–60 Gy are delivered to the normal tissue.
- It has been a mainstay treatment for oropharyngeal cancers for decades and excellent tumor control and functional results have been reported, especially with regard to swallowing and speech (**Figure 4.2**).[17-21]

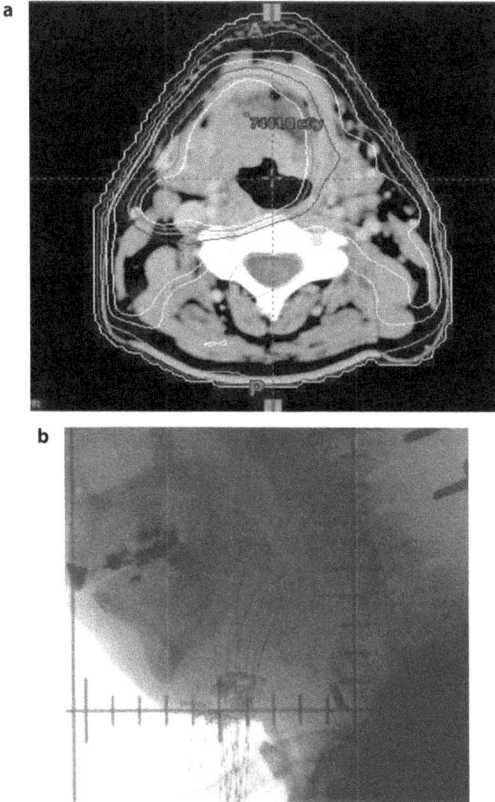

Figure 4.2 Example of Treatment of a Base of Tongue Cancer Treated with Concurrent Chemotherapy, IMRT, Brachytherapy, and Neck Dissection Example of 62-year-old male patient with a T2 N2bM0 base of tongue carcinoma treated with combined external-beam radiation and concurrent chemotherapy, brachytherapy implant, and planned neck dissection. External-beam radiation was delivered with intensity-modulated radiation with a reduced dose of 5940 cGy to the involved primary site and nodes with three cycles of cisplatin given on days 1, 22, and 43 of radiation followed by 20 Gy brachytherapy boost to the tongue base and neck dissection.

Surgery

- Surgery for tumors of the oropharynx traditionally required an open surgical approach in order to access the tumors in this region and to perform a meaningful resection.

- An open surgical approach to the oropharynx requires a mandibulotomy in order to swing the mandible laterally and gain access to the oropharynx.[22]

- When an open approach is used, this area must be reconstructed by transferring tissue using microvascular surgery.

- The radial forearm and anterolateral thigh free flaps remain the most common flaps for relining the oropharynx and reconstituting the volume loss of the base of tongue.

- If the patient has significant comorbidities or does not want to undergo the rigors of a microvascular reconstruction, a pectoralis major rotation flap can be utilized to reline the oropharynx and restore bulk to the base of the tongue.

- In recent years, transoral laser surgery has become increasingly popular for resecting tumors of the oropharynx.[23]

- This approach requires no external incisions or a mandibulotomy and therefore significantly decreases the morbidity of a surgical resection.

- Depending on the size of the initial tumor, patients may require a temporary tracheostomy for airway protection.

- Often this approach to tumors of the oropharynx allows for patients to be speaking and swallowing within a few days from surgery and the hospital stays are significantly shorter than those of the open approach.

- More recently, the DaVinci robot has been incorporated in transoral surgery to further enhance the ability to resect tumors while minimizing the morbidity associated with oropharyngeal surgery.[23]

- In general, small oropharyngeal lesions with a clinically negative neck or small-volume nodes represent the best candidates for primary resection and neck dissection.

- The primary advantage is that pathologic information can better tailor the need for radiation or chemoradiation.
- The potential disadvantage is that patients may be subjected to invasive procedures with marginal benefit, especially if they proceed to concurrent chemoradiation.

■ Treatment of Locally Advanced Resectable Disease: Stage III and IV

- The majority of patients with oropharynx cancer will present with stage III and IV disease and do require a multimodality approach that combines chemotherapy, radiation therapy, and surgery.
- For most advanced cases, primary chemoradiation is recommended to maximize organ and function preservation.
- Radiation alone provides suboptimal rates of local control in T3–4 lesions or patients with advanced N2–3 neck disease due to high rates of persistent disease after treatment compared to combined treatment.
- Neck dissection is often integrated up front in patients with high-volume nodal disease.
- Brachytherapy can be added to further boost dose to the primary site, and reduced external beam administered to normal tissues.
- With regard to primary chemoradiation, major strides have been achieved with the incorporation of altered fractionated radiation, chemotherapy, and biologic therapy.
- Altered fractionation radiation has been shown to improve outcomes over conventional radiation treatment (seven weeks of daily radiation therapy to deliver 70 Gy) by accelerating treatments (giving twice-a-day radiation treatment to shorten treatment time to six weeks and deliver 70 Gy)[24,25] or by hyperfractionated dose escalation (giving twice-a-day treatments over seven weeks to deliver 77–80 Gy).[26]
- Meta-analyses indicate a survival advantage of hyperfractionation with dose escalation compared to conventional fractionation.[27]

- Altered fractionated radiation is often considered in patients with stage III/IV disease who cannot undergo standard concurrent chemoradiation.
- Numerous overviews demonstrate the advantage of adding chemotherapy to radiation.[28,29]
- A meta-analysis by Monnerat concludes that concurrent chemotherapy offers an 8% survival benefit, induction chemotherapy 2%, and adjuvant therapy a 1% benefit.[28]
- The primary benefit of concurrent chemoradiation is improved locoregional control and organ preservation.[30]
- The standard chemotherapy regimen in a patient with good performance status is three doses of cisplatin at 100 mg/m2 given weeks 1, 4, and 7 of a standard course of radiotherapy.

Targeted Therapy

- In patients who are not candidates for concurrent chemoradiation, an important treatment alternative is a targeted therapy against the epidermal growth factor receptor.
- A monoclonal antibody directed against epidermal growth factor receptor, cetuximab, has been shown in a phase III trial to improve locoregional control and survival compared to radiation therapy alone.[30]
- Cetuximab is usually well tolerated and associated with high compliance during radiation therapy. It is considered in patients with impaired renal or hearing function and patients with compromised performance status.

Induction Chemotherapy

- Induction chemotherapy has been utilized to reduce tumor burden and predict successful treatment of tumors to organ preservation therapy.
- With regard to survival benefit, previous meta-analyses showed only a minor benefit of induction chemotherapy.[28]
- However, recent data show that the addition of docetaxel (Taxotere) to induction cisplatin/5-fluorouracil followed

by radiation or concurrent chemoradiation improves survival and locoregional control.[31,32]

▦ The choice of the combined modality program to be used is often dependent on the treating team and their experience. The options include:

1. Surgery followed by radiation therapy or chemoradiation. The use of surgical resection up front often entails open resection with unilateral or bilateral neck dissection followed by adjuvant radiation with or without chemotherapy.

2. Integration of reconstructive flaps is crucial toward maintenance of function and appearance.

3. Concurrent chemoradiotherapy. The use of concurrent chemoradiotherapy is considered by many to represent the standard of care when treating patients with locally advanced oropharynx cancer.

4. The agent that is studied the most is bolus cisplatin at 100 mg/m^2 to be given every three weeks during radiation.

   ▦ Patients who cannot tolerate this dose and schedule of platinum can be treated with weekly chemotherapy using one of the following regimens:

   • Weekly carboplatin and paclitaxel
   • Weekly cisplatin
   • Weekly cetuximab

▦ The benefit of chemotherapy is difficult to prove after age 70 based on meta-analysis of multiple trials in head and neck cancer and even though age is not used as a stratification factor in deciding on the use of chemotherapy, the treating oncologist needs to be aware of the effect of age on the overall morbidity and mortality in head and neck cancer.[33,34]

▦ Sequential chemoradiotherapy. The use of induction chemotherapy followed by radiation therapy or concurrent chemoradiotherapy has been extensively studied and does represent another option in treating patients with locally advanced disease.

   • The induction chemotherapy regimen that is the most widely used is TPF: Docetaxel, cisplatin, and continuous infusion 5 fluorouracil to be given every three weeks for a total of three cycles at the following doses:

- Cisplatin 100 mg/m^2 day 1
- Docetaxel 75 mg/m^2 day 1
- 5-fluorouracil 1000 mg/m^2 per day on days 1, 2, 3, and 4 via continuous infusion

- After three cycles of induction chemotherapy, patients are treated with chemoradiotherapy using weekly carboplatin at an area under the curve (AUC) 1.5.
- This intensive regimen should only be used in patients with an excellent performance status and a normal kidney and liver function.
- In trying to decide when to use concurrent chemoradiotherapy or sequential chemoradiotherapy, factors favoring the use of sequential chemoradiotherapy include:
  - Patients at high risk of distant metastasis such as those with high-volume N2 or N3 disease
  - Patient with T4 disease
  - Patients in need of immediate therapy
  - Patients in whom there is a high suspicion that distant metastasis has already occurred
  - Circumstances where a delay in starting radiotherapy is anticipated

■ Treatment of Locally Advanced Unresectable Disease

- For patients with unresectable disease, the same treatment modalities discussed previously are applicable with the exception of surgical resection.
- For these patients, surgery is not an option, and either chemoradiotherapy or sequential chemoradiotherapy should be employed.
- These patients have a worse prognosis than the resectable group with a cure rate of 25–40% at 5 years.

■ References

1. Dahlstrand HM, Dalinis T. Presence and influence of human papillomaviruses (HPV) in tonsillar cancers. *Adv Cancer Res.* 2005;93:59–89.

2. Gillison ML, Koch WM, Capone RB, et al. Evidence for a causal association between human papillomavirus and a subset of head and neck cancers. *J Natl Cancer Inst.* 2000;92(9):709–720.

3. Gillison ML, D'Souza G, Westra W, et al. Distinct risk factor profiles for human papillomavirus type 16-positive and human papillomavirus type 16-negative head and neck cancers. *J Natl Cancer Inst.* 2008;100(6):407–420.

4. Weinberger P, Yu Z, Haffty B, et al. Molecular classification identifies a subset of human papillomavirus—associated oropharyngeal cancers with favorable prognosis. *J Clin Oncol.* 2006;24(5)736–747.

5. Ang KK, Harris J, Wheeler R, et al. Human papillomavirus and survival of patients with oropharyngeal cancer. *N Engl J Med.* 2010;363(1):24–35.

6. Klussmann JP, Gultekin E, Weissenborn SJ, et al. Expression of p16 protein identifies a distinct entity of tonsillar carcinomas associated with human papillomavirus. *Am J Pathol.* 2003;162(3):747–753.

7. Rouviere H. *Anatomy of the Human Lymphatic System.* Ann Arbor, MI: Edward Brothers; 1938.

8. Mendenhall WM, Morris CB, Amdur RJ, et al. Definitive radiotherapy for tonsillar squamous cell carcinoma. *Am J Clin Oncol.* 2006;29(3):290–297.

9. Spanos WJ Jr, Shukovsky LJ, Fletcher GH. Time, dose and tumour volume relationships in irradiation of squamous cell carcinomas of the base of the tongue. *Cancer.* 1976;37:2591.

10. Amdur RJ, Mendenhall WM, Parsons JT, et al. Carcinoma of the soft palate treated with irradiation: analysis of results and complications. *Radiother Oncol.* 1987;9:185.

11. Fein DA, Mendenhall WM, Parsons JT, et al. Pharyngeal wall carcinoma treated with radiotherapy: impact of treatment technique and fractionation. *Int J Radiat Oncol Biol Phys.* 1993;26;751.

12. O'Sullivan B, Warde P, Grice B, et al. The benefits and pitfalls of ipsilateral radiotherapy in carcinoma of the tonsillar region. *Int J Radiat Oncol Biol Phys.* 2001;51(2):332–343.

13. Eisbruch A, Kim HM, Terrell JE, et al. Xerostomia and its predictors following parotid-sparing irradiation of head-and-neck cancer. *Int J Radiat Oncol Biol Phys.* 2001;50:332–343.

14. Chao KS, Deasy JO, Markman J, et al. A prospective study of salivary function sparing in patients with head-and-neck cancers receiving intensity-modulated or three dimensional radiation therapy: initial results. *Int J Radiat Oncol Biol Phys.* 2001;49:907–916.

15. Eisbruch, Schwartz M, Rasch C, et al. Dysphagia and aspiration after chemoradiotherapy for head-and-neck cancer: which

anatomic structures are affected and can they be spared by IMRT? *Int J Radiat Oncol Biol Phys.* 2004;60(5):1425–1439.

16. Huang K, Lee N, Xia P, et al. Intensity-modulated radiotherapy in the treatment of oropharyngeal carcinoma:a single institutional experience. *Int J Radiat Oncol Biol Phys.* 2003;57(S2):2303.

17. de Arruda FF, Puri DR, Zhung J, et al. Intensity-modulated radiation therapy for the treatment of oropharyngeal carcinoma: the Memorial Sloan-Kettering Cancer Center experience. *Int J Radiat Oncol Biol Phys.* 2006;64(2):363–373.

18. Pernot M, Malissard L, Taghian A, et al. Velotonsillar squamous cell carcinoma: 277 cases treated by combined external irradiation and brachytherapy—results according to extension, localization and dose rate. *Int J Radiat Oncol Biol Phys.* 1992;23:715–723.

19. Levendag PC, Teguh DN, Voet P, et al. Dysphagia disorders in patients with cancer of the oropharynx are significantly affected by the radiation therapy dose to the superior and middle constrictor muscle: a dose-effect relationship. *Radiother Oncol.* 2007;85(1):64–73.

20. Harrison LB, Zelefsky MJ, Sessions RB, et al. Base-of-tongue cancer treated with external beam irradiation plus brachytherapy: oncologic and functional outcome. *Radiology.* 1992;184:267–270.

21. Patton B, Hu K, Persky M, et al. *Survival and Toxicity Outcomes in Base of Tongue Cancer Treated with Brachytherapy Boost Combined with 2D or IMRT: A Ten year experience.* ASTRO; 2010, San Diego, CA.

22. Weber RS, Peters LJ, Wolf P, et al. Squamous cell carcinoma of the soft palate, uvula and anterior facial pillar. *Otolaryngol Head Neck Surg.* 1988;99:16.

23. Weinstein GS, O'Malley BW Jr, Cohen MA, et al. Transoral robotic surgery for advanced oropharyngeal carcinoma. *Arch Otolaryngol Head Neck Surg.* 2010;136(11):1079–1085.

24. Fu KK, Pajak TF, Trotti A, et al. A radiation therapy oncology group (RTOG) phase III randomized study to compare hyperfractionation and two variants of accelerated fractionation to standard fractionation radiotherapy for head and neck squamous cell carcinomas. First report of RTOG 9003. *Int J Radiat Oncol Biol Phys.* 2000;48(1):7–16.

25. Overgaard J, Hansen HS, Specht L, et al. Five compared with six fractions per week of conventional radiotherapy of squamous-cell carcinoma of head and neck: DAHANCA 6 and 7 randomised controlled trial. *Lancet.* 2003;362(9388):933–940.

26. Horiot JC, Le Fur R, N'Guyen T. Hyperfractionation versus conventional fractionation in oropharyngeal carcinoma: final

analysis of a randomized trial of the EORTC cooperative group of radiotherapy. *Radiother Oncol.* 1992;25:231–241.

27. Bourhis J, Overgaard J, Audry H, et al. Hyperfractionated or accelerated radiotherapy in head and neck cancer: a meta-analysis. *Lancet.* 2006;368(9538):843–854.

28. Monnerat C, Faivre S, Temam S, et al. End points for new agents in induction chemotherapy for locally advanced head and neck cancers. *Ann Oncol.* 2002;13(7):995–1006.

29. Pignon JP, Bourhis, J, Domenge, C, et al. Chemotherapy added to locoregional treatment for head and neck squamous-cell carcinomas: three meta-analyses of updated individual data. MACH-NC Collaborative Group. Meta-analysis of chemotherapy on head and neck cancer. *Lancet.* 2000;355:949–955.

30. Calais G, Alfonsi M, Bardet E, et al. Randomized trial of radiation therapy versus concomitant chemotherapy and radiation therapy for advanced-stage oropharynx carcinoma. *J Natl Cancer Inst.* 1999;91:2016–2081.

31. Bonner J, Harari P, Giralt J, et al. Radiotherapy plus cetuximab for squamous-cell carcinoma of the head and neck. *N Engl J Med.* 2006 Feb 9;354(6):567–578.

32. Vermorken JB, Remenar E, van Herpen C, et al. Cisplatin, fluorouracil, and docetaxel in unresectable head and neck cancer. *N Engl J Med.* 2007. 357(17):1695–1704.

33. Posner MR, Hershock DM, Blajman CR, et al. Cisplatin and fluorouracil alone or with docetaxel in head and neck cancer. *N Engl J Med.* 2007. 357(17):1705–1715.

34. Bourhis J, Le Maître A, Baujat B. Meta-Analysis of Chemotherapy in Head, Neck Cancer Collaborative Group; Meta-Analysis of Radiotherapy in Carcinoma of Head, Neck Collaborative Group; Meta-Analysis of Chemotherapy in Nasopharynx Carcinoma Collaborative Group. *Curr Opin Oncol.* 2007 May;19(3):188–194.

Larynx/Hypopharynx

■ Epidemiology

■ Larynx cancer represents the most common site of squamous cell carcinoma in the head and neck region with approximately 10,000 cases diagnosed each year (see **Figure 5.1**).

■ Risk factors include smoking, alcohol consumption, and gastroesophageal reflux disease.

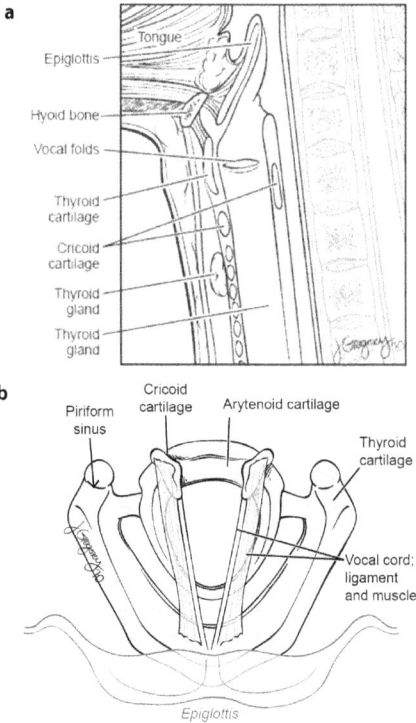

Figure 5.1 Anatomy of the Larynx and Hypopharynx
(a) Sagittal view. (b) Axial view.
Source: Courtesy of Jill K. Gregory, Continuum Health Partner.

- Presenting symptoms include hoarseness, dysphagia, otalgia, pain, nodal disease, and obstructive dyspnea.
- About 95% of all are squamous cell carcinoma; fewer than 5% are sarcoma, adenocarcinoma, lymphoma, or neuroendocrine tumors.
- Workup includes a physical exam, endoscopy with documentation of lesion extent, vocal cord mobility, and ruling out of synchronous primary sites.
- Computed tomography of the neck to evaluate cartilage invasion and nodal metastases.
- Positron emission tomography/computed tomography scan can be obtained to further refine staging and evaluate for distant disease. Dental evaluation especially if cervical nodal irradiation is planned.
  - Fluoride prophylaxis and ongoing surveillance of the patient posttreatment.
  - Dental extractions should be performed prior to radiation therapy and often require a 10-day to 2-week break prior to initiation of treatment.

■ Glottic Larynx Cancer

Early Stage

- Vocal cord lesions diagnosed in early stage are highly curable as they have a low propensity for nodal metastasis and can be managed with single-modality treatment.
- Surgery or radiation are considered for early stage lesions while most often a combination of chemotherapy, surgery, and radiation are considered for advanced lesions.
- For advanced lesions, multidisciplinary treatment is designed to maximize tumor cure, preserve organ function, address regional spread, and tailor treatment to patient's comorbidities and preference.
- Radiation therapy alone to the larynx offers excellent tumor control and organ function preservation.
- Current techniques entail simple lateral fields to deliver 63–65 Gy in 28–29 fractions over 5½ weeks (see **Figure 5.2**).
- The fields are typically 5 × 5 or 6 × 6 cm to encompass the vocal cords, subglottic area, and inferior aspect of the supraglottic larynx.

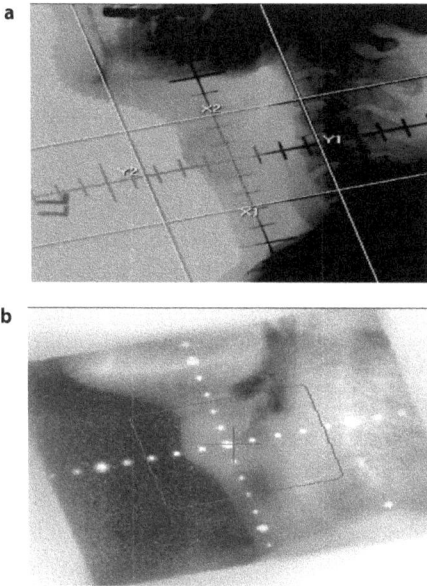

Figure 5.2 Early Stage Glottic Larynx Cancer Treatment
Treatment of early stage glottic larynx cancer focuses radiotherapy on the larynx only without coverage of the draining lymph nodes.

- The draining lymph nodes are not typically included in the radiation fields.
- Treatment to the larynx alone without elective nodal coverage spares treatment of the major salivary glands, mandible, and oropharynx/oral cavity.
- Treatment duration is best kept to less than 6 weeks of total time.
- For T2 lesions with impaired vocal cord mobility or subglottic extension, a hyperfractionated radiation schedule can improve local control, albeit with increased acute toxicity.
- For T1 and T2 lesions, local control is typically greater than 90% and 80%, respectively.[1]
- Laser excision and partial laryngectomy represent effective options to control disease, but voice quality may be suboptimal if a significant volume of the vocal fold needs to be removed or the anterior commissure is involved.[2]

- In general, small midvocal lesions are the best candidates for laser resection with preservation of voice.
- Laser excision is performed transorally without the need for any external incisions, and often the patient can be discharged home the same day as surgery.
- Oncologic results have been shown to be equally effective as radiation therapy with the added benefit of sparing the rest of the larynx from collateral damage.
- T1 and select T2 lesions are often surgically approached with a CO_2 laser resection.

Advanced Stage

- Total laryngectomy followed by postoperative radiation therapy once represented the standard of care for advanced glottic larynx cancers.
- However, the landmark Veterans Administration laryngeal trial demonstrated that organ preservation nonsurgical therapy was possible in 2/3 of patients who underwent induction chemotherapy followed by radiation without compromise of survival when compared to the control arm of total laryngectomy and postoperative radiation.[3]
- A subsequent randomized, intergroup trial of patients with primarily T2–3 tumors comparing the Veterans Administration regimen to concurrent chemoradiation or radiation alone demonstrated that concurrent chemoradiation is superior to the Veterans Administration induction regimen in improving larynx preservation (from 75% to 88%) and represents the current standard of care.[4]
- No difference in overall survival was noted among all three arms because of high surgical salvage rates.[5]
- Acute grade 3–4 toxicity, particularly mucositis, dermatitis, and nausea, was greater in patients undergoing concurrent treatment compared to patients in the other two arms.
- Thus, for patients with good performance status, radiation consisting of 7 weeks of daily radiation to deliver 70 Gy given concurrently with high-dose cisplatin at 100 mg/m^2 for three cycles is recommended.

- More intensive induction regimens consisting of three drugs Docetaxel (T), Cisplatinum (P), and 5-fluorouracil (F) TPF followed by chemoradiation or radiation alone are considered.[6]
- In patients who are debilitated and unable to tolerate standard chemotherapy, other options include radiation therapy alone or radiation therapy with a biologic therapy comprised of a monoclonal antibody targeting the epidermal growth factor receptor.
- If radiation alone is considered, then a course of altered fractionated radiation therapy may be considered with either hyperfractionation or accelerated therapy.[7,8]
- The patients excluded from the organ preserving chemoradiation studies are tumors that invaded cartilage and/or extended outside the larynx into soft tissues.
- The gold standard for these patients remains total laryngectomy.
- Superficial cartilage involvement is not considered a definitive reason to avoid larynx preservation. Organ preservation in these patients with chemoradiation is feasible.

T4 Disease

- For advanced T4 lesion with extensive disease invading thyroid cartilage or extending extralaryngeally, total laryngectomy followed by adjuvant radiation with possible concurrent chemotherapy is standard treatment.
- Patients with poor laryngopharyngeal function before treatment may be better served with primary resection with reconstruction and adjuvant radiation or chemoradiation.

■ Optimizing Patient Outcomes

- In order to optimize the chance for success from radiation therapy, patients must avoid smoking during treatment (smoking increases radiation resistance of the tumor) and be highly compliant with the radiation schedule, avoiding treatment delays totaling more than five days.

■ Patients should undergo supportive care evaluation with a speech/swallowing team, a nutritionist, pain management, and a psychosocial service team to help them cope with acute and chronic effects of treatment.

■ Acute and Chronic Side Effects

Acute Chemoradiation

■ Over a six-and-a-half-to-seven-weeks course of treatment, patients usually begin to experience morbidity from radiation during the third week of treatment consisting of dermatitis, mucus production, sore throat, hoarseness, dysphagia, fatigue, dysgeusia, and xerostomia.

■ By the second half of treatment as symptoms intensify, most patients require creams/emollients for skin care, medication to control mucus, narcotics for pain, change in diet to soft solids and liquid nutritional supplements, and antiemetic agents.

■ Gastrostomy tube placement maybe considered for patients not deemed strong enough to proceed through treatment.

■ If nausea is not properly addressed, patients may develop severe weight loss, which will impair their ability to heal as well as complete treatment.

Chronic

■ Patients will recover several weeks to several months after treatment and will typically be off medications by four to six weeks after treatment.

■ Important long-term side effects include fibrosis of the neck, dental caries from xerostomia, dysphagia, hypothyroidism, and xerostomia.

■ Supraglottic Larynx Cancer

■ Tumors located at other sites of the larynx (false vocal cords, arytenoids, epiglottis, aryepiglottic folds) require management of the neck even for early stage tumors as there is a higher proclivity for regional involvement regardless of stage.

- The primary tumor can spread into the paralaryngeal space, causing vocal cord fixation; and to the preepiglottic space with extension into the tongue base, through thyroid cartilage into the soft tissues outside of the larynx, and laterally into the hypopharynx.

Early Stage Lesions

- T1–2 lesions of the supraglottic larynx require management of the primary site with elective treatment of the draining lymph nodes at level II–IV.
- Similar to early stage vocal cord cancers, these tumors may be managed with single modality therapy.
- Radiation consists of 66–70 Gy to treat the primary site and elective neck therapy to a dose of 50–54 Gy.
- Surgery consists of vocal cord sparing surgery and neck dissection(s) and may be considered for patients with adequate pulmonary status and ability to rehabilitate.
- Transoral surgery and open partial laryngectomy are the surgical approaches that can be utilized to approach these tumors.

Advanced-Stage Lesions

- Advanced-stage lesions are managed very similarly to T3–4 glottic larynx cancers.
- Chemoradiation is recommended for patients with appropriate performance status and good baseline laryngopharyngeal function, while primary resection followed by adjuvant radiation or chemoradiation is recommended in disease with extralaryngeal spread or poor baseline function.

■ Subglottic Larynx Cancer

- Tumors located under the vocal cords are rare and clinically difficult to visualize even with endoscopy, requiring exam under anesthesia.
- Because of their occult nature, they often present with advanced lesions invading the trachea and soft tissues of the neck.

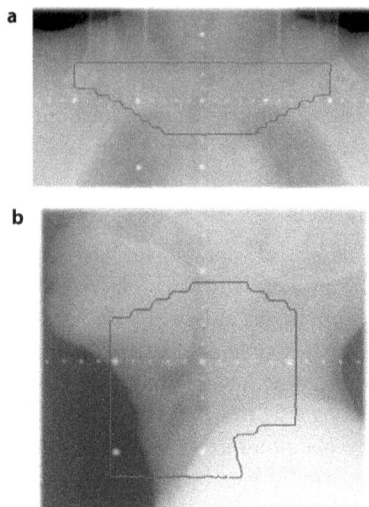

Figure 5.3 Supraglottic Larynx Cancer Treatment for Early T-Stage Disease
Treatment of early stage supraglottic larynx cancer requires treatment of the larynx and upper neck nodes (a) but also the low neck nodes (b).

- Such tumors are at risk for spreading to the inferior cervical nodal chains as well as the superior mediastinal nodes.
- The most common site of distant metastasis is the lung, which should be distinguished from a metachronous/synchronous primary site.
- Example of early stage glottic versus supraglottic larynx cancer treatment:
  a. Early stage glottic larynx cancer treatment requires treatment to the larynx alone (Figure 5.2).
  b. Supraglottic larynx cancer treatment for early T-stage disease requires treatment of the upper and lower cervical nodes (**Figure 5.3**).

■ Hypopharynx

- The hypopharynx represent a small subset of head and neck patients and has the lowest chance for cure due to its high proclivity for early nodal involvement, distant disease, and resistance to treatment.

- It is located in a crucial area of the laryngopharynx with all tumors potentially impacting on voice, swallowing, and breathing.

Treatment

- About 25% of all hypopharynx cancers present as early stage disease and are amenable to radiation therapy alone or larynx conservation procedures.
- The risk for nodal involvement is 30–40%, thus neck management is indicated.
- Local control varies between 47% and 90%, and five-year survival is 11–52%. In general, the best results are obtained with conventional fractionation to doses of > 65 Gy for T1 lesions and hyperfractionated radiation for T2 lesions.[9–11]
- For advanced stage lesions, laryngopharyngectomy followed by postoperative radiation with or without chemotherapy is standard treatment.
- Small tumors with nodal involvement and nonbulky T3 lesions may be considered for management with radiation therapy and chemotherapy.[12]
- In this setting, patients may be treated with upfront concurrent chemoradiation consisting of three doses of cisplatin with seven weeks of radiation therapy.
- Alternatively, induction chemotherapy with Docetaxel, Cisplatinum, and 5-fluorouracil TPF followed by radiation alone has been considered as well as an alternative to concurrent chemoradiation in an effort to minimize long-term swallowing complications from fibrosis.
- The addition of docetaxel (Taxotere) to cisplatinum/ 5-fluorouracil TPF followed by radiation increases larynx preservation.
- A French trial randomized 220 patients with hypopharynx or larynx cancer for whom total laryngectomy was indicated to either Docetaxel, Cisplatinum, and 5-fluorouracil, or Cisplatinum and 5-fluorouracil TPF or PF followed by conventional fractionated radiation to a dose of 70 Gy in seven weeks.
- Complete response was increased in the Docetaxel, Cisplatinum, and 5-fluorouracil TPF arm from 47% to 61% and at a median follow-up of 61 months, the 5-year

larynx preservation rate was increased from 51% to 74%. Five-year laryngoesophageal dysfunction-free survival was increased in the Docetaxel, Cisplatinum, and 5-fluorouracil TPF arm from 39% to 60%.

- Bulky T3 lesions and T4 lesions are best considered for up-front total laryngopharyngectomy followed by adjuvant therapy because tumor control and function preservation are suboptimal after nonsurgical therapy, and patients often have morbidity such as chronic aspiration due to poor swallowing.

■ Total Laryngectomy

- A total laryngectomy requires a large apron incision to allow access to the entire contents of the left and right neck.
- The visceral compartment of the neck is then separated from the great vessels and the entire larynx is removed by making mucosal incisions above the hyoid bone and vertically along the pharynx until the esophageal inlet is reached.
- Great care is taken to preserve as much nondiseased mucosal tissue as possible in order to optimized postlaryngectomy speech and swallowing function.
- The larynx is then detached from the trachea by transecting the trachea below the cricoid cartilage.
- A permanent stoma is created above the collarbones, and commonly a tracheoesophageal puncture is created so that a voice prosthesis can be placed for postlaryngectomy voice.
- If enough of the lining of the pharynx is preserved, a primary closure of the mucosa can be performed to reconstruct the pharynx.
- If the tumor extends far enough into the lining of the pharynx that a primary closure cannot be performed, a fasciocutaneous-free flap (radial forearm or anterolateral thigh flap) or a pectoral myocutaneous flap can be utilized to reconstruct the lining of the pharynx.
- These flaps can be tubed for circumferential defects or used as a patch for partial pharyngectomy defects.

▨ Adjuvant radiation with or without chemotherapy is usually recommended after resection. The decision of whether concurrent chemoradiation is needed is based on pathologic factors (see Chapter 3, "Oral Cavity Cancer").

▣ References

1. Le QT, Fu KK, Kroll S, et al. Influence of fraction size, total dose, and overall time on local control of T1-T2 glottic carcinoma. *Int J Radiat Oncol Biol Phys.* 1997;39(1):115–126.
2. Ogura JH, Biller HF, Weete R. Elective neck dissection for pharyngeal and laryngeal cancers: an evaluation. *Ann Oral Rhinol Laryngol.* 1971;8: 646.
3. Induction chemotherapy plus radiation compared with surgery plus radiation in patients with advanced laryngeal cancer. The Department of Veterans Affairs Laryngeal Cancer Study Group. *N Engl J Med.* 1991;324(24):1685–1690.
4. Forastiere AA, Goepfert H, Maor M, et al. Long-term results of Intergroup RTOG 91-11: a phase III trial to preserve the larynx—induction cisplatin/5-FU and radiation therapy versus concurrent cisplatin and radiation therapy versus radiation therapy. *J Clin Oncol.* 2006;24(18S): 5517.
5. Weber RS, Berkey BA, Forastiere A, et al. Outcome of salvage total laryngectomy following organ preservation therapy: the Radiation Therapy Oncology Group trial 91-11. *Arch Otolaryngol Head Neck Surg.* 2003;129(1):44–49.
6. Calais G, Debelleix C, Sire C. et al. Induction chemotherapy followed by radiation for larynx preservation, functional results of the Gortec 2000-01 randomized trial. Presented at the plenary session, Multidisciplinary Head and Neck Symposium; 2010; Phoenix, AZ.
7. Overgaard J, Hansen HS, Specht L, et al. Five compared with six fractions per week of conventional radiotherapy of squamous-cell carcinoma of head and neck: DAHANCA 6 and 7 randomised controlled trial. *Lancet.* 2003;362(9388):933–940.
8. Fu KK, Pajak TF, Trotti A, et al. A radiation therapy oncology group (RTOG) phase III randomized study to compare hyperfractionation and two variants of accelerated fractionation to standard fractionation radiotherapy for head and neck squamous cell carcinomas: first report of RTOG 9003. *Int J Radiat Oncol Biol Phys.* 20001;48(1):7–16.
9. Amdur RJ, Mendenhall WM, Stringer SP, et al. Organ preservation with radiotherapy for T1-T2 carcinoma of the piriform sinus. *Head Neck.* 2001;23:353.

10. Garden AS, Morrison WH, Ang KK, et al. Hyperfractionated radiation in the treatment of squamous cell carcinomas of the head and neck. *Int J Radiat Oncol Biol Phys.* 1995;31:493.
11. Johansen LV, Grau C, Overgaard J. Hypopharyngeal squamous cell carcinoma—treatment results in 138 consecutively admitted patients. *Acta Oncol.* 2000;39:529.
12. Lefebvre JL, Chevalier D, Luboinski B, et al. Larynx preservation in pyriform sinus cancer: preliminary results of a European Organization of Research and Treatment of Cancer phase III trial. *J Natl Cancer Inst.* 1996;88:890.

Sinonasal Carcinoma

◼ Anatomy

- The nasal fossa and paranasal sinuses consist of a labyrinth of well-aerated, mucosal lined, and interconnected cavities (see **Figure 6.1**).
- The nasal fossa is divided into two separate chambers by the nasal septum.
- There are three paired turbinates within the nasal fossa, which further subdivides the nasal vault from superior to inferior.
- The ethmoid sinuses are made up of a network of bony partitions that drain into the nasal fossa.
- The maxillary sinuses are the largest of the paranasal sinuses, and they reside within the body of the maxilla.
- The sphenoid sinus is located posterior to the nasal fossa and superior to the adenoids.

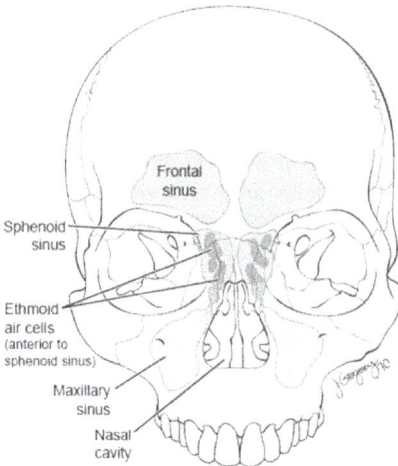

Figure 6.1 Anatomic Illustration of the Subsites Comprising the Sinonasal Area
Source: Courtesy of Jill K. Gregory, Continuum Health Partners.

- The frontal sinus is located in the frontal bone and is divided into two unequal halves by the intersinus septum.

■ Incidence and Risk Factors

- Malignancies of the paranasal sinuses are rare; there are 2000 newly diagnosed cases of carcinoma of the paranasal sinuses in the United States annually.
- Men are more commonly affected by these malignancies.
- Approximately 60–70% of these malignancies occur in the maxillary sinuses, and 20–30% occur in the nasal cavity proper.[1–3]
- Risk factors include exposure to nickel dust, mustard gas, Thorotrast, isopropyl oil, chromium, dichlorodiethyl sulfide, and wood dust.
- Wood dust has been shown to increase the risk of squamous cell carcinoma 21 times and the risk of adenocarcinoma 874 times.[4–6]
- Interestingly, preliminary studies show that human papilloma virus and Epstein-Barr virus infection may be an early event in the transformation of inverting papilloma to a malignant lesion.[7–9]
- The most common histologies include:
  - Malignant inverting papilloma
  - Squamous cell carcinoma
  - Adenoid cystic carcinoma
  - Adenocarcinoma
  - Malignant melanoma
  - Sinonasal neuroendocrine tumors
  - Esthesioneuroblastoma
  - Verrucous carcinoma
  - Lymphoma
  - Minor salivary gland malignancies (mucoepidermoid carcinoma, carcinoma ex pleomorphic)
  - Metastatic malignant tumors

■ Signs and Symptoms

- Tumors within the nasal vault or the paranasal sinuses present with nasal airway obstruction, epistaxis, pain, and nasal discharge.

- They can originate in any of the paranasal sinuses or the nasal cavity proper and often remain silent or are mistakenly treated as an infectious or inflammatory condition, with a consequent delay in the diagnosis.
- More ominous signs are facial paresthesias, proptosis, and diplopia.

Workup

- The history and physical should focus on evidence of nasal obstruction, epistaxis, pain, anosmia, hyposmia, foul odor headaches, chronic infection, and pain.
- The examination must include palpation of the neck for metastasis as well as a nasal endoscopy to visually evaluate for ulcerative, polypoid masses of the nasal fossa, which may be biopsied endoscopically in the majority of cases.
- Computed tomography scan without contrast is used to evaluate the extent of local disease and plan for an endoscopic biopsy.
- Magnetic resonance imaging is extremely helpful in examining for perineural invasion, skull base involvement, intracranial extension, orbital invasion, and invasion of the masticator and/or parapharyngeal spaces by a tumor.
- Additionally, magnetic resonance imaging is very helpful in differentiating between tumor and retained secretions within the sinuses.

■ Staging

Maxillary Sinus

Primary Tumor (T)

- T1: Tumor limited to maxillary sinus mucosa with no erosion or destruction of bone.
- T2: Tumor causing bone erosion or destruction including extension into the hard palate and/or the middle of the nasal meatus, except extension to the posterior wall of the maxillary sinus and pterygoid plates.
- T3: Tumor invades any of the following: bone of the posterior wall of maxillary sinus, subcutaneous tissues,

floor or medial wall of orbit, pterygoid fossa, or ethmoid sinuses.

- ▪ T4a: Tumor invades anterior orbital contents, skin of cheek, pterygoid plates, infratemporal fossa, cribriform plate, or sphenoid or frontal sinuses.
- ▪ T4b: Tumor invades any of the following: orbital apex, dura mater, brain, middle cranial fossa, cranial nerves other than maxillary division of trigeminal nerve (V2), nasopharynx, or clivus.

Nasal Cavity and Ethmoid Sinus
Primary Tumor (T)

- ▪ T1: Tumor restricted to any one subsite, with or without bony invasion.
- ▪ T2: Tumor invading two subsites in a single region or extending to involve an adjacent region within the naso-ethmoidal complex, with or without bony invasion.
- ▪ T3: Tumor extends to invade the medial wall or floor of the orbit, maxillary sinus, palate, or cribriform plate.
- ▪ T4a: Tumor invades any of the following: anterior orbital contents, skin of nose or cheek, minimal extension to anterior cranial fossa, pterygoid plates, or sphenoid or frontal sinuses.
- ▪ T4b: Tumor invades any of the following: orbital apex, dura mater, brain, middle cranial fossa, cranial nerves other than V2, nasopharynx, or clivus.

Regional Lymph Nodes (N)

- ▪ N1: Metastasis in a single ipsilateral lymph node, 3 cm or less in greatest dimension
- ▪ N2: Metastasis in a single ipsilateral lymph node, more than 3 cm but 6 cm or less in greatest dimension; or in multiple ipsilateral lymph nodes, 6 cm or less in greatest dimension; or in bilateral or contralateral lymph nodes, 6 cm or less in greatest dimension
- ▪ N2a: Metastasis in a single ipsilateral lymph node more than 3 cm but 6 cm or less in greatest dimension
- ▪ N2b: Metastasis in multiple ipsilateral lymph nodes, 6 cm or less in greatest dimension

- N2c: Metastasis in bilateral or contralateral lymph nodes, 6 cm or less in greatest dimension
- N3: Metastasis in a lymph node more than 6 cm in greatest dimension

Kadish Staging for Esthesioneuroblastoma

- *Stage A*: The tumor is limited to the nasal fossa.
- *Stage B*: The tumor extends to the paranasal sinuses.
- *Stage C*: The tumor extends beyond the paranasal sinuses.

■ Treatment

- For early stage lesions, surgery may be used to grossly resect tumors and radiation added if adverse pathologic features are present.
- In advanced cases where the orbit is at risk or if gross total resection is uncertain, preoperative chemoradiation followed by resection may be utilized to enhance the chance for organ preservation if there is limited orbital invasion or to decrease the chance of a positive margin in those with extensive intracranial extension.
- Advanced lesions that are unresectable may be treated with definitive chemoradiation.
- Surgical resection can be approached endoscopically or open.
- Endoscopy provide a high resolution, magnified view of the anatomy and allow the surgeons to visualize this area in ways that were not possible previously.
- Small tumors that can be approached endoscopically are removed without the need for the traditional open surgery incisions (transfacial incisions).
- Over the past 10 years, surgeons have become increasingly comfortable with endoscopic resection of tumors and have pushed the limits of resection to include tumors that require resection of the skull base.

■ Goals of Surgical Resection and Reconstruction

Details of Endoscopic/Open Surgery

- Reconstruction of an ablative defect from an open resection of a paranasal sinus malignancy should be considered.

- When a tumor of the paranasal sinuses is approached surgically, the extent of the resection and the patient's motivation for rehabilitation determine the reconstructive approach applied.

Palate

- Tumors that require resection of the hard palate often leave patients with a large oronasal or oroantral fistula.
- These can be obturated with a dental prosthesis or patched closed with a soft-tissue flap.
- Hard-tissue flaps (i.e., fibular-free flaps) are most commonly reserved for patients who will ultimately undergo a dental rehabilitation with osseointegrated implants.

Orbit

- If resection of the tumor requires resection of part or all of the orbital floor, this structure must be meticulously reconstructed to prevent the globe from migrating inferiorly and posteriorly resulting in diplopia as well as a poor cosmetic outcome.
- Additionally, if the globe must be exenterated, the orbit can be reconstructed with a soft-tissue flap to fill the volume deficit.
- If there is a plan for an ocular reconstruction, a maxillofacial prosthodontist must be consulted. Osseointegrated implants can be extremely helpful in fixating an ocular prosthesis.

■ Complications

The complications of treating a malignant sinonasal tumor surgically are:

1. *Epistaxis*: Usually originates from the anterior or posterior ethmoid arteries, or the sphenopalatine artery
2. *Cerebrospinal fluid leak*: This includes clear rhinorrhea, salty taste in mouth, and meningitis
3. *Epiphora*: Due to obstruction of the lacrimal outflow tract.
4. *Diplopia*: Commonly occurs if the orbital floor is resected during the ablation.

■ Goals of Definitive Chemoradiation for Advanced Disease

■ The use of intensity modulated radiation therapy to treat sinonasal tumors has significantly decreased the incidence of severe toxicity due to the ability to shape radiation away from critical surrounding structures such as the optic nerve, chiasm, brainstem, spinal cord, and brain.[10]

■ The incidence of complications is related to the total dose delivered to the tumor bed and the adjacent structures.

■ The brainstem, optic nerve, chiasm, and brain have radiation tolerances of 54–60 Gy, which may be readily achieved in the majority of postoperative cases where a dose of 60–63 Gy is delivered.

■ However, in the definitive setting, doses of 66–70 Gy are required to eradicate gross disease and special care must be taken to limit late toxicity.

■ The key to successful treatment requires detailed imaging of the tumor with magnetic resonance imaging and positron emission tomography/computed tomography.

■ If tumor involves the orbital apex, chiasm skull bases, or extends intracranially, then the risk of brain necrosis and blindness must be weighed against the probability of tumor control.

■ Outcomes after definitive chemoradiation using intensity modulated radiation therapy show local control rates of about 60%.[11,12]

■ References

1. Bridger GP, Mendelsohn MS, Baldwin M, Smee R. Paranasal sinus cancer. *Aust N Z J Surg.* 1991;61:290–294.
2. Golabek W, Drop A, Golabek E, Morshed K. Site of origin of paranasal sinus malignancies. *Pol Merkur Lekarski.* 2005;19:413–414.
3. Larsson LG, Martensson G. Carcinoma of the paranasal sinuses and the nasal cavities: a clinical study of 379 cases treated at Radiumhemmet and the Otolaryngologic Department of Karolinska Sjukhuset, 1940–1950. *Acta Radiol.* 1954;42:149–172.
4. Klintenberg C, Olofsson J, Hellquist H, Sokjer H. Adenocarcinoma of the ethmoid sinuses: a review of 28 cases

with special reference to wood dust exposure. *Cancer*. 1984;54:482–488.

5. Luce D, Gerin M, Leclerc A, Morcet JF, Brugere J, Goldberg M. Sinonasal cancer and occupational exposure to formaldehyde and other substances. *Int J Cancer*. 1993;53:224–231.

6. Leclerc A, Martinez Cortes M, Gerin M, Luce D, Brugere J. Sinonasal cancer and wood dust exposure: results from a case-control study. *Am J Epidemiol*. 1994;140:340–349.

7. Katori H, Nozawa A, Tsukuda M. Markers of malignant transformation of sinonasal inverted papilloma. *Eur J Surg Oncol*. 2005;31:905-911.

8. McKay SP, Gregoire L, Lonardo F, Reidy P, Mathog RH, Lancaster WD. Human papillomavirus (HPV) transcripts in malignant inverted papilloma are from integrated HPV DNA. *Laryngoscope*. 2005;115:1428–1431.

9. Ott G, Kalla J, Ott MM, Muller-Hermelink HK. The Epstein-Barr virus in malignant non-Hodgkin's lymphoma of the upper aerodigestive tract. *Diagn Mol Pathol*. 1997;6:134–139.

10. Hoppe BS, Wolden SL, Zelefsky ML, et al. Postoperative intensity-modulated radiation therapy for cancers of the paranasal sinuses, nasal cavity and lacrimal glands: technique, early outcomes and toxicity. *Head Neck*. 2008;30:925–932.

11. Blanco AI, Chao KS, Ozyigit G, et al. Carcinoma of paranasal sinuses: long-term outcomes with radiotherapy. *Int J Radiat Oncol Biol Phys*. 2004;59:51–58.

12. Chen AM, Daly ME, Bucci MK, et al. Carcinomas of the paranasal sinuses and nasal cavity treated with radiotherapy at a single institution over five decades: are we making improvement? *Int J Radiat Oncol Biol Phys*. 2007;69(1):141–147.

Management of Thyroid Carcinoma

■ Introduction

- Thyroid cancer is a result of gene mutations that lead to the uncontrolled growth of either follicular cells or para-follicular cells.
- Thyroid cancer can range in virulence from the indolent, well-differentiated forms of thyroid cancer (papillary and follicular) to the rapidly growing aggressive anaplastic thyroid cancer.
- Estimated new cases and deaths from thyroid cancer in the United States in 2010[1]:
  - *New cases*: 44,670
  - *Deaths*: 1,690
- In the United States, the incidence of thyroid cancer increased 82% from 1995 to 2005.[2]

■ Anatomy

The thyroid gland is a brownish-colored gland that resides on the trachea, just below the cricoid cartilage (see **Figure 7.1**). It is a butterfly-shaped structure with a variety of important structures lying within close proximity. Its vascular supply is composed of a superior thyroid artery and vein, middle thyroid vein, and inferior thyroid artery and vein on either side of the gland. The paired recurrent laryngeal nerves run along the posterior of the gland and enter the cricothyroid joint to innervate the vocal cords. Additionally, there are paired superior laryngeal nerves that run along the medial aspect of the superior portion of the lateral lobes. The superior laryngeal nerves innervate the cricothyroid muscles to control pitch of the voice. Finally, there are four parathyroid glands that reside along the posterolateral surface of the thyroid gland. These glands are vital to maintain calcium homeostasis.

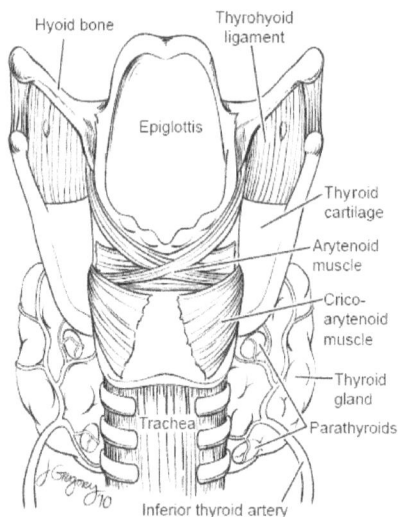

Figure 7.1 Posterior View of the Thyroid Gland and Its Relation to Surrounding Larynx and Hypopharynx
Source: Courtesy of Jill K. Gregory, Continuum Health Partners.

■ Risk Factors

- Family history of thyroid cancer
- History of radiation exposure:
  - Prior history of head and neck irradiation (i.e., radiation for Hodgkin's disease or head and neck cancer)
  - Occupational radiation exposure
  - Radiation exposure from nuclear reactor accident
- Male gender
- Age > 70
- Age < 20
- Lateral neck mass
- Evidence of invasion of surrounding structures on imaging

■ Signs and Symptoms

- Rapid growth of an existing thyroid nodule
- Pain
- Change in voice
- Dysphagia

Workup

▣ Ultrasound of the thyroid and cervical lymphatics (levels II-VI bilaterally).

▣ A fine-needle aspiration of the primary thyroid mass and any suspicious lymph nodes is performed.

■ Staging

Separate stage groupings are recommended for papillary or follicular, medullary, and anaplastic (undifferentiated) carcinoma.

TNM Classification

Papillary or Follicular Thyroid Cancer

Younger than 45 Years[3]

▣ Stage I
  • Any T, any N, M0
▣ Stage II
  • Any T, any N, M1

Age 45 years and older

▣ Stage I
  • T1, N0, M0
▣ Stage II
  • T2, N0, M0
▣ Stage III
  • T3, N0, M0
  • T1, N1a, M0
  • T2, N1a, M0
  • T3, N1a, M0
▣ Stage IVA
  • T4a, N0, M0
  • T4a, N1a, M0
  • T1, N1b, M0
  • T2, N1b, M0
  • T3, N1b, M0
  • T4a, N1b, M0
▣ Stage IVB
  • T4b, any N, M0

- Stage IVC
  - Any T, any N, M1

Medullary Thyroid Cancer

- Stage I
  - T1, N0, M0
- Stage II
  - T2, N0, M0
- Stage III
  - T3, N0, M0
  - T1, N1a, M0
  - T2, N1a, M0
  - T3, N1a, M0
- Stage IVA
  - T4a, N0, M0
  - T4a, N1a, M0
  - T1, N1b, M0
  - T2, N1b, M0
  - T3, N1b, M0
  - T4a, N1b, M0
- Stage IVB
  - T4b, any N, M0
- Stage IVC
  - Any T, any N, M1

Anaplastic Thyroid Cancer

All anaplastic carcinomas are considered stage IV.
- Stage IVA
  - T4a, any N, M0
- Stage IVB
  - T4b, any N, M0
- Stage IVC
  - Any T, any N, M1

Papillary and Follicular Thyroid Cancer

- Stage I papillary thyroid cancer
  - Localized to the thyroid gland and is 2 cm or less in size.
  - There often are multiple foci of this disease within the gland.

- Stage II papillary thyroid cancer
  - Tumor that has spread distantly in patients younger than 45 years
  - Tumor that is larger than 2 cm but 4 cm or smaller and is limited to the thyroid gland in patients older than 45 years.
- Stage III papillary thyroid cancer
  - Patients must be older than 45 years
  - The tumor is larger than 4 cm and is limited to the thyroid or with minimal extrathyroidal extension
  - Positive lymph nodes limited to the pretracheal, para-tracheal, or prelaryngeal/delphian nodes
- Stage IV papillary thyroid cancer
  - Patients must be older than 45 years
  - Extension beyond the thyroid capsule to the soft tissues of the neck, cervical lymph node metastases, or distant metastases
- Stage I follicular thyroid cancer
  - Localized to the thyroid gland and is 2 cm or less in size
- Stage II follicular thyroid cancer
  - In patients < 45 years the tumor has spread distantly.
  - In patients > 45 years the tumor is larger than 2 cm but less than 4 cm and is limited to the thyroid gland.
- Stage III follicular thyroid cancer
  - Patients must be > 45 years
  - Tumor is > 4 cm and limited to the thyroid or with minimal extrathyroidal extension, or positive lymph nodes limited to the pretracheal, paratracheal, or prelaryngeal/delphian nodes
- Stage IV follicular thyroid cancer
  - Patients must be older than 45 years.
  - Extension beyond the thyroid capsule to the soft tissues of the neck, cervical lymph node metastases, or distant metastases.
  - Follicular carcinomas more commonly have blood vessel invasion and tend to metastasize hematogenously to the lungs and to the bone rather than through the lymphatic system.

■ Hürthle cell carcinoma
  ● Hürthle cell carcinoma is a variant of follicular carcinoma with a similar prognosis and should be treated in the same way as equivalent stage non-Hürthle cell follicular carcinoma.[1]

Medullary Thyroid Cancer

■ Stage 0 medullary thyroid cancer
  ● Clinically occult disease detected by provocative biochemical screening
■ Stage I medullary thyroid cancer
  ● Tumor < 2 cm
■ Stage II medullary thyroid cancer
  ● Tumor > 2 cm but < 4 cm
■ Stage III medullary thyroid cancer
  ● Tumor > 4 cm with minimal extrathyroidal extension
  ● Primary tumor < 4 cm with metastases limited to the pretracheal, paratracheal, or prelaryngeal/delphian lymph nodes.
■ Stage IV medullary thyroid cancer is divided into:
  ● Stage IVA (potentially resectable with or without lymph node metastases [for T4a] but without distant metastases)
  ● Stage IVB (locally unresectable with or without lymph node metastases but no distant metastases)
  ● Stage IVC (distant metastases)

Anaplastic Thyroid Cancer

All patients are considered to have stage IV disease.

■ Treatment

Papillary and Follicular Thyroid Cancer

1. Total thyroidectomy plus removal of involved lymph nodes or other sites of extrathyroidal disease.
2. If there is evidence of lymph node involvement, a cervical lymphadenectomy is performed.
3. I-131 ablation following total thyroidectomy if the tumor demonstrates uptake of this isotope.

4. Utilized in the majority of differentiated thyroid cancers and improves locoregional control and survival.

5. Typical prescribed dose is 100–200 mCi.

6. Pretreatment uptake scans to determine if those with tumors may benefit and for dosing consideration.

7. External-beam radiation therapy is used selectively and provides primarily a locoregional control benefit.

8. It is considered if I-131 uptake by the tumor is poor for stage III and IV disease or in patients over 60 with adverse pathologic features such as recurrent disease, close or positive margins, soft-tissue extension especially into the tracheal-esophageal area, extracapsular extension, or multiple nodes.

9. External-beam radiation is typically delivered after I-131 ablation in I-131 avid tumors.

10. In metastatic disease, consideration should be given to enrollment in a clinical trial with a tyrosine kinase inhibitor.

11. Recently, b-raf inhibitors such as sorafenib have shown promise[4] and a large phase III placebo-controlled study is ongoing.

Medullary Thyroid Cancer

1. Patients with medullary thyroid cancer should be treated with a total thyroidectomy, unless there is evidence of distant metastasis.

2. In patients with clinically palpable medullary carcinoma of the thyroid, the incidence of microscopically positive nodes is more than 75%; routine central and bilateral modified neck dissections have been recommended.[5]

3. When cancer is confined to the thyroid gland, the prognosis is excellent.

4. External beam radiation therapy has been used to improve locoregional control and may be considered in patients with multiple high-risk features such as positive margins, multiple nodes, and extracapsular nodal extension.

5. It has been used for palliation of locally recurrent tumors, without evidence that it provides any survival advantage.[6]

6. Radioactive iodine has no place in the treatment of patients with medullary thyroid cancer.
7. Palliative chemotherapy:
   - Palliative chemotherapy has been reported to produce occasional responses in patients with metastatic disease.[7–10]
   - No single drug regimen can be considered standard.
   - Some patients with distant metastases will experience prolonged survival and can be managed expectantly until they become symptomatic.
   - Recently there have been significant advances reported with the use of tyrosine kinase inhibitors that target the RET oncogene.
   - A phase III study recently reported with vandetanib versus placebo showed a significant improvement in progression-free survival with vandetanib.[11]
   - Another agent of interest is XL-184, which also targets vascular endothelial growth factor and RET, and an international phase III, placebo controlled study is ongoing.[12]

Anaplastic Thyroid Cancer

1. Tracheostomy is frequently necessary to relieve or prevent breathing difficulty, which can be produced by mass effect or by vocal cord paralysis.
2. If the disease is confined to the local area, which is rare, total thyroidectomy is warranted to reduce symptoms.[13,14]
3. External-beam radiation therapy is used in conjunction with radiosensitizing chemotherapy such as doxorubicin or taxanes to maximize locoregional control.
4. Radiation is given in an accelerated hyperfractionated regimen to address the rapid repopulation of the tumor.
5. Anaplastic thyroid cancer is not responsive to I-131 therapy.
6. Approximately 30% of patients achieve a partial remission with doxorubicin.[15]
7. The combination of doxorubicin and cisplatin appears to be more active than doxorubicin alone and has been reported to produce more complete responses.[16]

Treatment Options Under Clinical Evaluation

▪ The combination of chemotherapy and radiation therapy in patients following complete resection may provide prolonged survival but has not been compared to any one modality alone.[17,18]

Recurrent Thyroid Cancer

▪ Patients with recurrent differentiated carcinoma are reevaluated for salvage resection and maximal I-131 radioablation.

▪ There are single-institutional reports of successful use of salvage radiation therapy for patients with unresectable cancer.

▪ Intensity-modulated radiation therapy is currently utilized to maximize radiation dose delivery with sparing of the spinal cord and swallowing structures.

▪ References

1. American Cancer Society: *Cancer Facts and Figures 2010.* Atlanta, GA: American Cancer Society; 2010.
2. Libutti SK. Understanding the role of gender in the incidence of thyroid cancer. *Cancer J.* 2005;11:104–105.
3. Thyroid. In: *American Joint Committee on Cancer: AJCC Cancer Staging Manual.* 6th ed. New York, NY: Springer; 2002:77–87.
4. Gupta-Abramson V, Troxel AB, Nellore A, et al. Phase II trial of sorafenib in advanced thyroid cancer. *J Clin Oncol.* 2008;26(29):4714–4719.
5. Moley JF, DeBenedetti MK. Patterns of nodal metastases in palpable medullary thyroid carcinoma: recommendations for extent of node dissection. *Ann Surg.* 1999;229:880–887; discussion 7–8.
6. Brierley JD, Tsang RW. External radiation therapy in the treatment of thyroid malignancy. *Endocrinol Metab Clin North Am.* 1996;25(1):141–157.
7. Shimaoka K, Schoenfeld DA, DeWys WD, et al. A randomized trial of doxorubicin versus doxorubicin plus cisplatin in patients with advanced thyroid carcinoma. *Cancer.* 1985;56(9):2155–2160.
8. De Besi P, Busnardo B, Toso S, et al. Combined chemotherapy with bleomycin, Adriamycin, and platinum in advanced thyroid cancer. *J Endocrinol Invest.* 1991;14(6): 475–480, 1991.

9. Wu LT, Averbuch SD, Ball DW, et al. Treatment of advanced medullary thyroid carcinoma with a combination of cyclophosphamide, vincristine, and dacarbazine. *Cancer.* 1994;73(2):432–436.

10. Orlandi F, Caraci P, Berruti A, et al. Chemotherapy with dacarbazine and 5-fluorouracil in advanced medullary thyroid cancer. *Ann Oncol.* 1994;5(8):763–765.

11. Wells SA, Robinson BG, Gagel RF, et al. Vandetanib (VAN) in locally advanced or metastatic medullary thyroid cancer (MTC): a randomized, double-blind phase III trial (ZETA). *J Clin Oncol.* 2010;28(15s):suppl; abstr 5503.

12. Kurzrock R, Cohen EE, Sherman SI, et al. Long-term results in a cohort of medullary thyroid cancer (MTC) patients (pts) in a phase I study of XL184 (BMS 907351), an oral inhibitor of MET, VEGFR2, and RET. *J Clin Oncol.* 2010;28(15s):suppl; abstr 5502.

13. Goldman JM, Goren EN, Cohen MH, et al. Anaplastic thyroid carcinoma: long-term survival after radical surgery. *J Surg Oncol.* 1980;14(4):389–394.

14. Aldinger KA, Samaan NA, Ibanez M, et al. Anaplastic carcinoma of the thyroid: a review of 84 cases of spindle and giant cell carcinoma of the thyroid. *Cancer.* 1978;41(6):2267–2275.

15. Carling T, Udelsman R. Thyroid tumors. In: DeVita VT Jr, Hellman S, Rosenberg SA, eds. *Cancer: Principles and Practice of Oncology.* 7th ed. Philadelphia, PA: Lippincott Williams & Wilkins; 2005:1502–1519.

16. Shimaoka K, Schoenfeld DA, DeWys WD, et al. A randomized trial of doxorubicin versus doxorubicin plus cisplatin in patients with advanced thyroid carcinoma. *Cancer.* 1985;56(9):2155–2160.

17. Haigh PI, Ituarte PH, Wu HS, et al. Completely resected anaplastic thyroid carcinoma combined with adjuvant chemotherapy and irradiation is associated with prolonged survival. *Cancer.* 2001;91(12):2335–2342.

18. De Crevoisier R, Baudin E, Bachelot A, et al. Combined treatment of anaplastic thyroid carcinoma with surgery, chemotherapy, and hyperfractionated accelerated external radiotherapy. *Int J Radiat Oncol Biol Phys.* 2004;60(4):1137–1143.

Cancer of the Nasopharynx

■ Epidemiology

- Nasopharyngeal carcinoma (NPC) is an endemic disease in southern China, northern Africa, and the Mediterranean basin.[1,2]
- It is rare in the United States and typically occurs in people from endemic areas.[2,3]
- The median age of presentation is 40–50 years, which is significantly younger than that of other head and neck cancers.[1]

Etiology

- Unlike squamous cell carcinomas at other sites in the head and neck, the etiology of nasopharynx carcinomas is strongly associated with Epstein-Barr virus (EBV) based on serologic and molecular markers.[4]
- Carcinogens related to diet (salted fish high in nitrosamine), poor hygiene, poor ventilation, smoking, and use of nasal balms have been implicated.[5,6]
- Serologic markers showing active EBV infection have been developed taking advantage of the presence of EBV in the tumor.
- All serologic markers of NPC have been based on the detection of antibodies to EBV[7] or on the detection of plasma EBV DNA.[8]
- Tumor markers may be useful for early detection, diagnosis, prognostication, and monitoring of treatment response.

■ Anatomy

- The nasopharynx is a cuboidal cavity located behind the choanae of the nasal cavity.

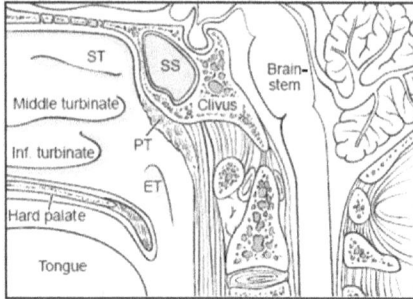

Figure 8.1 Anatomy of the Nasopharynx
Note the relation of the nasopharynx to the nasal cavity, clivus, sphenoid sinus, and oropharynx.
Source: Jill K. Gregory, Continuum Health Partners.

- It is comprised of two lateral walls, through which the eustachian tubes enter, and a roof that slopes downward toward the posterior pharyngeal wall down to the level of the uvula (see **Figure 8.1**).
- The most common site of origin of nasopharyngeal carcinoma lies posterior to the eustachian tube in a mucosal fold called Rosenmüller's fossa. Multiple structures surrounding the nasopharynx may be invaded by tumor including the clivus, parapharyngeal space near the masticatory muscles, and multiple foramina containing cranial nerves, arteries, and veins.

■ Diagnosis

- Diagnosis is made by pathologic confirmation, usually by biopsy of the nasopharynx or lymph node.
- Nearly all nonkeratinizing tumors, including differentiated and undifferentiated subtypes, will show EBV viral infection, best detected by fluorescent in situ hybridization analysis for EBV viral genome constituents in the neoplastic cells.

■ Signs and Symptoms

- Patients most commonly present with a painless neck mass in over one third, while other common manifestations include hearing loss or ear drainage in about one quarter and nasal bleeding or obstruction.

- Nasal symptoms including breathing obstruction, epistaxis, and discharge can occur.
- A small proportion of patients may present with cranial nerve deficit, most commonly involving the cranial nerves VI (diplopia) and V (numbness in V2 area most commonly).
- Patients may also present with facial pain, headaches, or neck discomfort.
- Proptosis will occur when cancer invades through the posterior portion of the orbit.
- Trismus is an indication of pterygoid muscle invasion.
- The majority of patients with NPC present with locoregionally advanced disease, and at least one fifth will have occult distant metastases.[9]
- Sites of predilection for metastatic spread most commonly include in order of greatest frequency: bone, lung, and liver.

■ Staging

The current staging system is the seventh edition of the American Joint Committee on Cancer staging[10] and represents the outcome of an evolution of 20 different systems and an international consensus of different staging systems used by the International Union Against Cancer system[11] (**Table 8.1**).

■ Management Strategies

- Nasopharyngeal carcinoma is a highly radio- and chemosensitive cancer that can be treated with high rates of locoregional control.
- Radiation therapy is able to cover the large areas of potential locoregional spread including bilateral cervical and retropharyngeal nodes as well as the parapharyngeal area, neural foramina, and paranasal sinuses.
- Advances in radiation delivery with intensity-modulated radiation therapy (IMRT), imaging, integration of

Table 8.1   AJCC Nasopharynx Staging Seventh Edition (2009)

T-Stage

T1: Tumor confined to the nasopharynx.

T2: Tumor extends to soft tissues.

T2a: Tumor extends to the oropharynx and/or nasal cavity without parapharyngeal extension.

T2b: Tumor with parapharyngeal extension.

T3: Tumor involves bony structures and/or paranasal sinuses.

T4: Tumor with intracranial extension or involvement of the cranial nerves, infratemporal fossa, hypopharynx, orbit, or masticator space.

Nodal

Regional nodal staging is unique for nasopharynx cancers compared to other head and neck squamous cell cancers:

N1: Unilateral cervical nodes and/or unilateral or bilateral retropharyngeal nodes 6 cm or less in greatest dimension without supraclavicular fossa involvement.

N2: Bilateral cervical nodes 6 cm or less in greatest dimension without supraclavicular fossa involvement.

N3: Nodes greater than 6 cm or involvement of the supraclavicular fossa.

N3a: Greater than 6 cm

N3b: Extension to the supraclavicular fossa.

Seventh Edition Staging

0:	Tis	N0	M0
I:	T1	N0	M0
II:	T2	N1	M0
	T1-2	N1	M0
III:	T1	N2	M0
	T2	N2	M0
	T3	N1-2	M0
IVa:	T4	N0-2	M0
IVb:		Any N3	M0
IVc:			Any M1

Source: Edge SB, Byrd DR, Compton CC, eds. *AJCC Cancer Staging Handbook.* 7th ed. New York, NY: Springer, 2010, Chapter 5, pages 69–70.

chemotherapy, standardization of an internationally agreed upon staging system, improvement of multidisciplinary care, and increased scientific exchange have led to significant advances in tumor control and quality of life.

▪ In general, patients with early stage tumors are amenable to treatment with radiation therapy alone with high rates of locoregional control, while those with T3–T4 lesions or significant nodal disease require more intensive chemoradiation treatment as outcomes with radiation therapy alone lead to higher rates of locoregional failure and distant metastases.

▪ For the latter group, multiple large trials testing the addition of chemotherapy show that the most effective treatment occurs when chemotherapy is delivered concurrently with radiation therapy.

▪ Brachytherapy and stereotactic radiosurgery have been used as boost treatment in the primary setting and as salvage therapy for patients with recurrent disease after standard radiation.

▪ In the latter setting, role of surgical salvage is an important consideration, especially in patients with localized disease.

▪ Radiation Technique

▪ Radiation treatment of nasopharynx cancer is best done with IMRT due to the proximity of tumors to critical structures including the spinal cord, brainstem, temporal lobes, and optic pathways, as well as structures important for quality of life and function such as masticatory/constrictor muscles, temporomandibular joint, salivary glands, and cochlea.

▪ These tumors often wrap around the brainstem in a concave manner as they spread into the parapharyngeal space, as well as intracranially through the skull base and foramina and along nerves.

▪ With IMRT, dose painting, in which differential doses to various target volumes are delivered simultaneously, is possible.

- Typically, doses of 66–70 Gy are delivered to areas of gross disease while lower doses (50–60 Gy) are delivered for areas at risk for occult disease.[12]

Dose Prescription

- The standard radiation dose prescribed to the primary site in nasopharyngeal cancer in most centers is 70 Gy over seven weeks.
- Doses of 66–70 Gy are given to involved nodes, and clinically uninvolved nodes typically receive 50 Gy in five weeks while intermediate risk areas for subclinical disease receive 60 Gy.

■ Early Stage Disease

Radiation Therapy Only

- Early stage patients represent less than 10% of all nasopharynx patients and may be treated with radiation therapy alone.
- Outcomes after radiation alone have shown generally good locoregional control rates for early stage tumors but suboptimal outcomes for locoregionally advanced tumors. After conventional radiation, local control is obtained in 75–95% for T1–2 compared to 44–80% for T3–4 tumors.[13-16]
- Improvement in disease control in early stage patients has been obtained by either dose escalation with brachytherapy or improved conformal technique.
- Moreover, with conformal techniques, improved function preservation of salivary glands, hearing, and overall quality of life have been demonstrated.

■ Brachytherapy

- For early T-stage tumors, boost using brachytherapy offers an opportunity to adequately cover the tumor with higher doses but avoid increased toxicity of additional external-beam radiation.[15,17]
- Typically, external-beam doses of 60–66 Gy are combined with brachytherapy doses of 12–18 Gy.[18]

■ Toxicity

■ The primary acute complications during external-beam radiation include mucositis, odynophagia, lymphedema, alteration of taste, xerostomia, fatigue, loss of appetite, dermatitis, alopecia, serous otitis media, and thrush.[19]

■ Long-term toxicities include xerostomia, lymphedema, fibrosis, osteoradionecrosis, soft-tissue necrosis, cranial neuropathy, carotid artery stenosis, temporal lobe necrosis, pharyngeal stricture, dysphagia, feeding tube dependence, trismus, otitis media, tympanic membrane perforation, deafness, hypopituitarism, and dental caries.[20]

■ Chemotherapy Management Strategies

Chemotherapy for Locoregionally Advanced Disease

■ Although excellent outcomes are obtained for treatment of early stage disease with radiotherapy alone, 20–60% of patients with advanced stage disease experience locoregional failure after radiotherapy alone[21] and high rates of distant metastases[22] with five-year overall survival of 28–56%.[21,23,24]

■ Cisplatin-based regimens have been found to be the most effective, and multiple phase III trials have been reported for both endemic and nonendemic nasopharynx cancer populations.[25,26]

■ Meta-analysis of 8 randomized trials with 1753 patients comparing chemotherapy and radiation to radiation therapy alone reported a hazard ratio of 0.82 (p = 0.006) favoring chemotherapy and corresponding to a 6% absolute five-year survival benefit.[27]

■ Concurrent chemotherapy provided an absolute event-free survival benefit of 10% at five years.

■ Induction chemotherapy improved event-free survival (HR = 0.82 [CI 0.67–0.97]) but not overall survival (HR = 0.99 [0.8–1.21]).

■ In the United States, the standard of care is concurrent chemoradiation with cisplatin chemotherapy and radiation followed by three cycles of adjuvant chemotherapy comprised of 5-fluorouracil and cisplatin.[25]

- The basis for such treatment is the landmark phase III randomized Intergroup Study 0099, which demonstrated that when compared to radiation alone, the addition of three cycles of CDDP (100 mg/m^2 q three weeks) to radiation therapy (70 Gy/seven weeks) followed by adjuvant CDDP/5-fluorouracil (80 mg/m^2 and 1000 mg/m^2 × four days, respectively) improved three-year locoregional control (from 59% to 86%) and decreased incidence of distant metastases (from 35% to 13%), which translated into an approximate 30–40% increase in three-year progression-free (69% vs 24%, $p < 0.001$) and overall survival (76% vs 46%, $p < 0.001$).
- The worst grade ¾ acute toxicity was increased in the chemoradiation arm (76% vs 50%) with a higher incidence of grade ¾ leukopenia and vomiting.
- Compliance to the planned regimen was compromised as only 63% were able to complete all three cycles of concurrent cisplatin with an additional 23% able to complete two concurrent cycles.
- Only 60% of patients received two to three planned cycles of adjuvant chemotherapy.
- Alternative schedules used outside of the United States have included weekly cisplatin (40 mg/m^2) with radiation alone without adjuvant chemotherapy and induction chemotherapy followed by chemoradiation.[26]

IMRT and Concurrent Chemoradiation

- IMRT has been widely adopted due to its superior ability to conform dose around the tumor and spare normal structures, resulting in excellent locoregional control and improvement in quality of life and function preservation.[12,28]
- Locoregional control is obtained in over 90% even in patients with advanced T3–4 or nodal disease with survival at 3–4 years of 80–90%.
- The improved dose conformality translates into preservation of quality of life and organ function.
- The amelioration of chronic xerostomia, the most common quality of life complaint after head and neck irradiation affecting the sense of comfort, taste, dental hygiene, and swallowing is well studied.

- Both objective (salivary flow measurement, standardized toxicity scores and sialo-scintigraphy) and patient validated subjective data have been established.[29–31]
- Other important structures to be spared include the cochlea, optic pathways, brainstem, spinal cord, cranial nerves, masticator muscles, and nausea center.
- Patients receiving conformal therapy experienced a clinically significant improvement in global quality of life, pain, speech, xerostomia, appetite, social eating, feeling ill, and dental health compared to patients treated with older techniques.[32]

■ Follow-up

Secondary Primary Tumors

- In contrast to other head and neck sites with the high incidence of secondary malignancies, the incidence is markedly lower after treatment for NPC.
- The incidence of secondary malignancies with a cumulative incidence of about 5–6% at five years primarily involve the aerodigestive tract.[33]

■ Salvage of Recurrent Disease

- Locoregionally recurrent disease after previous radiation therapy presents a challenging situation that requires multidisciplinary evaluation.
- Multiple surgical and radiation approaches are feasible salvage options particularly for the early stage recurrences.
- With advanced disease, options are usually limited to external-beam radiation techniques with integration of chemotherapy.
- Neck dissection is routinely incorporated in patients with resectable nodal recurrence.

■ External-Beam Reirradiation

- When local failure occurs, the chance for local control with subsequent treatment varies widely, with reported five-year control rates of 15–60%.[34–36]

- Prognostic factors important for local control and survival that are consistently reported from single institutional series include the stage of the recurrent tumor (T1–2 have more favorable outcomes), interval from previous radiation treatment (more than two-year interval from previous radiation), and whether the chronology suggests persistent versus recurrent disease.
- In general, for patients undergoing reirradiation, doses of > 60 Gy are required for with external-beam treatment.[34,37,38] The best salvage treatment must be individually tailored.
- Toxicity after salvage reirradiation may include fatal bleeding, mucosal necrosis, fibrosis, trismus, cranial neuropathy, temporal lobe necrosis, or osteoradionecrosis.[39]

■ Nasopharyngectomy

- With modern imaging, improved surgical technique, and supportive care, salvage nasopharyngectomy represents an important salvage option.
- Retrospective series report local control of 40–67% with best outcomes for early stage patients.[40-43]
- Multiple surgical approaches are considered depending on tumor location.
- Subtotal nasopharyngectomy can be undertaken via a transpalatal approach with centrally located small tumors, with a maxillary swing approach for more extensive tumors and anterolateral approach with facial translocation for advanced tumors.
- An anterior and/or middle fossa resection is indicated when the tumor extends superiorly to involve the infratemporal fossa or cavernous sinus.
- Surgical complications may include carotid artery injury, pharyngeal plexus palsy, osteomyelitis, palatal fistula, trismus, nasal regurgitation, dysphagia, and infection.

■ Chemotherapy for Recurrent and Metastatic Disease

- NPC is highly chemosensitive, and there have been multiple phase II trials demonstrating response rates of

50–90% to first-line combination chemotherapy, all of which contain platinum.[44,45]

▪ The choice of chemotherapy regimen is currently based more on toxicity profile and reported response rates from phase II trials.

▪ Current options of first-line chemotherapy will be cisplatin in combination with infusional 5-fluorouracil, paclitaxel, or gemcitabine.

▪ Newer chemotherapeutic agents demonstrating activity for NPC include irinotecan, capecitabine, docetaxel, vinorelbine, and oxaliplatin.[46-49]

▪ Incorporation of biologic agents targeting the epidermal and vascular endothelial growth factors remain to be defined.

▪ Long-Term Survivors After Chemotherapy for Metastatic Disease

▪ Several retrospective series have reported long-term survivors after systemic chemotherapy in metastatic NPC with survival over 36 months after achieving complete response to chemotherapy.[50]

▪ Patients with lung metastases only had a more favorable survival outcome after systemic chemotherapy compared with patients with other sites of failure.[51]

▪ Hence an aggressive approach to manage metastatic NPC patients with a good performance status is recommended, especially if the metastasis is confined to the intrathoracic site.

▪ References

1. Ho JH. An epidemiologic and clinical study of nasopharyngeal carcinoma. *Int J Radiat Oncol Biol Phys.* 1978;4(3-4):182–198.
2. Wenig BM. Nasopharyngeal carcinoma. *Ann Diagn Pathol.* 1999;3(6):374–385.
3. Marks JE, Phillips JL, Menck HR. The National Cancer Data Base report on the relationship of race and national origin to the histology of nasopharyngeal carcinoma. *Cancer.* 1998;83(3):582–588.
4. Raab-Traub N. Epstein-Barr virus in the pathogenesis of NPC. *Semin Cancer Biol.* 2002;12(6):431–441.

5. Buell P. The effect of migration on the risk of nasopharyngeal cancer among Chinese. *Cancer Res.* 1974;34(5):1189–1191.

6. Huang DP. Epidemiology and aetiology. In:. Van Hasselt AG, ed. *Nasopharyngeal Carcinoma.* Hong Kong: The Chinese Free Press; 1991:23–35.

7. Henle G, Henle W. Epstein-Barr virus-specific IgA serum antibodies as an outstanding feature of nasopharyngeal carcinoma. *Int J Cancer.* 1976;17(1):1–7.

8. Lo YM, Chan LY, Lo KW, et al. Quantitative analysis of cell-free Epstein-Barr virus DNA in plasma of patients with nasopharyngeal carcinoma. *Cancer Res.* 1999;59(6): 1188–1191.

9. Geara FB, Sanguineti G, Tucker SL, et al. Carcinoma of the nasopharynx treated by radiotherapy alone: determinants of distant metastasis and survival. *Radiother Oncol.* 1997;43(1):53–61.

10. Edge SB, Byrd DR, Compton CC, et al. (2009) American Joint Committee on Cancer, American Cancer Society. *AJCC cancer staging manual.* 7th ed. New York, NY: Springer: Berlin Heidelberg.

11. Lee AW, Foo W, Law SC, et al. Staging of nasopharyngeal carcinoma: from Ho's to the new UICC system. *Int J Cancer.* 1999;84(2): 179–187.

12. Lee N, Xia P, Quivey JM, et al. Intensity-modulated radiotherapy in the treatment of nasopharyngeal carcinoma: an update of the UCSF experience. *Int J Radiat Oncol Biol Phys.* 2002;53(1):12–22.

13. Mesic JB, Fletcher GH, Goepfert H. Megavoltage irradiation of epithelial tumors of the nasopharynx. *Int J Radiat Oncol Biol Phys.* 1981;7(4): 447–453.

14. Lee AW, Poon YF, Foo W, et al. Retrospective analysis of 5037 patients with nasopharyngeal carcinoma treated during 1976–1985: overall survival and patterns of failure. *Int J Radiat Oncol Biol Phys.* 1992;23(2):261–270.

15. Vikram B, Mishra UB, Strong EW, et al. Patterns of failure in carcinoma of the nasopharynx: I. Failure at the primary site. *Int J Radiat Oncol Biol Phys.* 1985;11(8):1455–1459.

16. Wang CC, Meyer JE. Radiotherapeutic management of carcinoma of the nasopharynx: an analysis of 170 patients. *Cancer.* 1971;28(3):566–570.

17. Qin DX, Hu YH, Yan JH, et al. Analysis of 1379 patients with nasopharyngeal carcinoma treated by radiation. *Cancer.* 1988;61(6):1117–1124.

18. Levendag PC, Lagerwaard FJ, Noever I, et al. Role of endocavitary brachytherapy with or without chemotherapy in cancer of the nasopharynx. *Int J Radiat Oncol Biol Phys.* 2002;52(3):755–768.

19. Marcial VA, Hanley JA, Chang C, et al. Split-course radiation therapy of carcinoma of the nasopharynx: results of a national collaborative clinical trial of the Radiation Therapy Oncology Group. *Int J Radiat Oncol Biol Phys.* 1980;6(4):409–414.

20. Lee AW, Law SC, Ng SH, et al. Retrospective analysis of nasopharyngeal carcinoma treated during 1976–1985: late complications following megavoltage irradiation. *Br J Radiol.* 1992;65(778):918–928.

21. Lee AW, Law SC, Foo W, et al. Nasopharyngeal carcinoma: local control by megavoltage irradiation. *Br J Radiol.* 1993;66(786):528–536.

22. Chan AT, Teo PM, Leung TW, et al. The role of chemotherapy in the management of nasopharyngeal carcinoma. *Cancer.* 1998;82(6):1003–1012.

23. Chu AM, Flynn MB, Achino E, et al. Irradiation of nasopharyngeal carcinoma: correlations with treatment factors and stage. *Int J Radiat Oncol Biol Phys.* 1984;10(12): 2241–2249.

24. Wang DC, Cai WM, Hu YH, et al. Long-term survival of 1035 cases of nasopharyngeal carcinoma. *Cancer.* 1988;61(11): 2338–2341.

25. Al-Sarraf M, LeBlanc M, Giri PG, et al. Chemoradiotherapy versus radiotherapy in patients with advanced nasopharyngeal cancer: phase III randomized Intergroup study 0099. *J Clin Oncol.* 1998;16(4):1310–1317.

26. Chan AT, Teo PM, Ngan RK, et al. Concurrent chemotherapy-radiotherapy compared with radiotherapy alone in locoregionally advanced nasopharyngeal carcinoma: progression-free survival analysis of a phase III randomized trial. *J Clin Oncol.* 2002;20(8):2038–2044.27.

27. Baujat B, Audry H, Bourhis J, et al. Chemotherapy in locally advanced nasopharyngeal carcinoma: an individual patient data meta-analysis of eight randomized trials and 1753 patients. *Int J Radiat Oncol Biol Phys.* 2006;64(1):47–56.

28. Kam MK, Teo PM, Chau RM, et al. Treatment of nasopharyngeal carcinoma with intensity-modulated radiotherapy: the Hong Kong experience. *Int J Radiat Oncol Biol Phys.* 2004;60(5):1440–1450.

29. Eisbruch A, Kim HM, Terrell JE, et al. Xerostomia and its predictors following parotid-sparing irradiation of head-and-neck cancer. *Int J Radiat Oncol Biol Phys.* 2001;50(3): 695–704.

30. Chao KS, Deasy JO, Markman J, et al. A prospective study of salivary function sparing in patients with head-and-neck cancers receiving intensity-modulated or three-dimensional radiation therapy: initial results. *Int J Radiat Oncol Biol Phys.* 2001;49(4):907–916.

31. Liu WS, Kuo HC, Lin JC, et al. Assessment of salivary function change in nasopharyngeal carcinoma treated by parotid-sparing radiotherapy. *Cancer J.* 2006;12(6):494–500.

32. Fang FM, Tsai WL, Chen HC, et al. Intensity-modulated or conformal radiotherapy improves the quality of life of patients with nasopharyngeal carcinoma: comparisons of four radiotherapy techniques. *Cancer.* 2007;109(2):313–321.

33. Kong L, Lu JJ, Hu C, et al. The risk of second primary tumors in patients with nasopharyngeal carcinoma after definitive radiotherapy. *Cancer.* 2006;107(6):1287–1293.

34. Wang CC. Re-irradiation of recurrent nasopharyngeal carcinoma—treatment techniques and results. *Int J Radiat Oncol Biol Phys.* 1987;13(7):953–956.

35. Lee AW, Law SC, Foo W, et al. Retrospective analysis of patients with nasopharyngeal carcinoma treated during 1976–1985: survival after local recurrence. *Int J Radiat Oncol Biol Phys.* 1993;26(5):773–782.

36. Leung TW, Tung SY, Sze WK, et al. Salvage radiation therapy for locally recurrent nasopharyngeal carcinoma. *Int J Radiat Oncol Biol Phys.* 2000;48(5):1331–1338.

37. Syed AM, Puthawala AA, Damore SJ, et al. Brachytherapy for primary and recurrent nasopharyngeal carcinoma: 20 years' experience at Long Beach Memorial. *Int J Radiat Oncol Biol Phys.* 2000;47(5):1311–1321.

38. Chua DT, Sham JS, Kwong PW, et al. Linear accelerator-based stereotactic radiosurgery for limited, locally persistent, and recurrent nasopharyngeal carcinoma: efficacy and complications. *Int J Radiat Oncol Biol Phys.* 2003; 56(1):177–183.

39. Li JC, Hu CS, Jiang GL, et al. Dose escalation of three-dimensional conformal radiotherapy for locally recurrent nasopharyngeal carcinoma: a prospective randomised study. *Clin Oncol (R Coll Radiol).* 2006;18(4):293–299.

40. King WW, Ku PK, Mok CO, et al. Nasopharyngectomy in the treatment of recurrent nasopharyngeal carcinoma: a twelve-year experience. *Head Neck.* 2000;22(3):215–222.

41. Fee WE Jr, Moir MS, Choi EC, et al. Nasopharyngectomy for recurrent nasopharyngeal cancer: a 2- to 17-year follow-up. *Arch Otolaryngol Head Neck Surg.* 2002;128(3): 280–284.

42. Wei WI, Ho CM, Yuen PW, et al. Maxillary swing approach for resection of tumors in and around the nasopharynx. *Arch Otolaryngol Head Neck Surg.* 1995;121(6):638–642.

43. Chua DT, Sham JS, Hung KN, et al. Predictive factors of tumor control and survival after radiosurgery for local failures of nasopharyngeal carcinoma. *Int J Radiat Oncol Biol Phys.* 2006;66(5):1415–1421.

44. Ma BB, Tannock IF, Pond GR, et al. Chemotherapy with gemcitabine-containing regimens for locally recurrent or metastatic nasopharyngeal carcinoma. *Cancer.* 2002;95(12):2516–2523.
45. Yeo W, Leung TW, Chan AT, et al. A phase II study of combination paclitaxel and carboplatin in advanced nasopharyngeal carcinoma. *Eur J Cancer.* 1998;34(13):2027–2031.
46. Wang CC, Chang JY, Liu TW, et al. Phase II study of gemcitabine plus vinorelbine in the treatment of cisplatin-resistant nasopharyngeal carcinoma. *Head Neck.* 2006;28(1):74–80.
47. Poon D, Chowbay B, Cheung YB, et al. Phase II study of irinotecan (CPT-11) as salvage therapy for advanced nasopharyngeal carcinoma. *Cancer.* 2005;103(3):576–581.
48. Chua DT, Kwong DL, Sham JS, et al. A phase II study of ifosfamide, 5-fluorouracil and leucovorin in patients with recurrent nasopharyngeal carcinoma previously treated with platinum chemotherapy. *Eur J Cancer.* 2000;36(6):736–741.
49. McCarthy JS, Tannock IF, Degendorfer P, et al. A phase II trial of docetaxel and cisplatin in patients with recurrent or metastatic nasopharyngeal carcinoma. *Oral Oncol.* 2002;38(7):686–690.
50. Fandi A, Bachouchi M, Azli N, et al. Long-term disease-free survivors in metastatic undifferentiated carcinoma of nasopharyngeal type. *J Clin Oncol.* 2000;18(6):1324–1330.
51. Hui EP, Leung SF, Au JS, et al. Lung metastasis alone in nasopharyngeal carcinoma: a relatively favorable prognostic group. A study by the Hong Kong Nasopharyngeal Carcinoma Study Group. *Cancer.* 2004;101(2):300–306.

CHAPTER 9

Recurrent Head and Neck Cancer

■ Introduction

- Many patients with head and neck cancer will suffer from recurrent or metastatic disease.
- The recurrence can be divided into local/regional recurrence and/or distant recurrence.
- Local regional recurrence refers to the cancer returning at the primary site and/or in the neck.
- Distant recurrence refers to the cancer returning at remote sites from the primary such as in the lungs, liver, and bone.

■ Treatment Approaches with Chemotherapy or Biologic Therapies

- The first question that is often asked when faced with a recurrence is whether the patient can be treated with a curative intent with surgery and/or reirradiation.
- This can sometimes be achieved when a patient has a local and or regional recurrence.
- Patients with distant metastatic disease are typically not curable and are treated for palliation with chemotherapy.

Treatment with Palliative Chemotherapy or Biologic Therapy

- This section describes the palliative treatment of patients with recurrent disease where a curative option is not possible.
- Performance status plays a key role in deciding on the use of chemotherapy in these patients. Patients with a poor performance status might not be candidates for palliative chemotherapy, and hospice care is appropriate.
- When deciding to use chemotherapy in these patients, there are many options available,[1] and they depend on

the prior chemotherapy regimens received and the length of time that has elapsed since chemotherapy was last used.

- In general, the same chemotherapy regimen is not used if the recurrence occurred within one year of receiving chemotherapy, and patients are considered resistant to those drugs.
- Platinum-based chemotherapy has been the standard first-line treatment for recurrent or metastatic squamous-cell carcinoma of the head and neck.
- Cisplatin or carboplatin is often combined with 5-fluorouracil, assuming the patient has not recently received these drugs.

Platinum-Based Regimens

- A phase III randomized study comparing cisplatin (P) and 5-fluorouracil (F) (PF) as single agents and in combination for advanced squamous-cell carcinoma of the head and neck found a higher overall response rate for the combination (32%) compared to cisplatin (17%) or 5-fluorouracil (13%) alone.
- Response was associated with good performance status.
- Median time to progression was less than 2.5 months, and there was no significant difference in median survival (5.7 months) among the groups.[2]
- The Southwest Oncology Group study conducted a randomized comparison of cisplatin plus fluorouracil and carboplatin plus fluorouracil versus methotrexate (MTX) in advanced squamous-cell carcinoma of the head and neck.[3]
- All three treatment regimens were well tolerated.
- However, both hematologic and nonhematologic toxicities were significantly greater with cisplatin plus 5-fluorouracil compared with MTX. The complete and partial response rates were 32% for cisplatin plus 5-fluorouracil, 21% for carboplatin plus 5-fluorouracil, and 10% for MTX.
- The comparison of cisplatin plus 5-fluorouracil to MTX was statistically significant, and the comparison of

carboplatin plus 5-fluorouracil to MTX was of borderline statistical significance.

- Median response durations and median survival times were similar for all three treatment groups.
- Performance status was associated significantly with survival.
- The authors concluded that combination chemotherapy resulted in improved response rates but was associated with an increased toxicity and no improvement in overall survival.
- It should be noted, though, that even though survival might not be improved with two drugs versus one, a higher response rate can be beneficial in these patients when it translates into less pain and better swallowing and this should be taken into consideration.

Role of Taxane-Based Chemotherapy

- Recently, the addition of docetaxel to PF chemotherapy has resulted in a survival benefit in patients with new diagnosis of head and neck cancer.
- This is based on two randomized phase III studies (TAX 323 and TAX 324) comparing docetaxel, cisplatin, and 5-fluorouracil TPF to cisplatin and 5-fluorouracil PF.[4,5]
- The TPF regimen has not been studied in the recurrent setting, and its use would not be recommended.
- The same could be said about cisplatin/docetaxel, a regimen that is much easier to give compared to PF or TPF since 5-fluorouracil continuous infusion is not required.
- This regimen results in a high response rate but its effect on overall survival is not known.[6,7]
- Docetaxel[8] as a single agent can be used in patients with recurrent disease and has shown response rates that vary depending on the setting in which they are used—first line versus subsequent lines of therapy.

Biologic Therapy Targeting the Epidermal Growth Factor Receptor

- Recently, cetuximab, an epidermal growth factor receptor inhibitor, has become available for patients with recurrent head and neck cancer and as a single agent in patients with platinum refractory disease.[10]

- As a single agent, cetuximab has a modest activity with about a 15% response.[10]

- Cetuximab has also been studied in combination with platinum and 5-fluorouracil in the first-line recurrent setting (i.e., the patient has a recurrence but has not received chemotherapy yet for that recurrence), in a randomized phase III study—the EXTREME Study.[11]

- In this study, patients with untreated recurrent or metastatic squamous-cell carcinoma of the head and neck received cisplatin (100 mg/m^2 on day 1) or carboplatin (at an area under the curve of 5 mg per milliliter per minute, as a one-hour intravenous infusion on day 1) plus fluorouracil (at a dose of 1000 mg/m^2 per day for four days) every three weeks for a maximum of six cycles or the same chemotherapy plus cetuximab (at a dose of 400 mg/m^2 initially, as a two-hour intravenous infusion, then 250 mg/m^2, as a one-hour intravenous infusion per week) for a maximum of six cycles.

- Patients with stable disease who received chemotherapy plus cetuximab continued to receive cetuximab until disease progression or unacceptable toxic effects.

- This study showed that adding cetuximab to platinum-based chemotherapy with fluorouracil significantly prolonged the median overall survival from 7.4 months in the chemotherapy-alone group to 10.1 months in the group that received chemotherapy plus cetuximab.

- The addition of cetuximab prolonged the median progression-free survival time from 3.3 to 5.6 months and increased the response rate from 20% to 36%.

- Skin toxicity related to cetuximab was also common.

- It can be concluded from this study that the addition of cetuximab to PF chemotherapy improved overall survival when given as first-line treatment in patients with recurrent or metastatic squamous-cell carcinoma of the head and neck.

- Testing for epidermal growth factor receptor expression for treatment purposes is not recommended at this stage for head and neck cancer patients.

Summary of Palliative Systemic Therapy

- When faced with a recurrent disease situation, the options for chemotherapy are the following:
  1. Platinum (cisplatin or carboplatin) with or without 5-fluorouracil
  2. Platinum (cisplatin or carboplatin) with a taxane (docetaxel or paclitaxel)
  3. Single-agent cetuximab
  4. Single-agent methotrexate
  5. Single-agent taxanes (docetaxel or paclitaxel)
  6. Cetuximab, in combination with platinum and 5-fluorouracil
  7. Enrollment in a clinical trial
- Enrollment in a clinical trial is essential to advance the field, and it is highly recommended to refer patients with recurrent disease to enroll in clinical trials in an effort to identify new agents and new targets that would ultimately help improve the dismal response rates and survival encountered in these patients.

■ Salvage Surgery

- When a patient presents with a local recurrence, usually the first option is a surgical salvage procedure.
- If the recurrence is local and small, the surgeon usually returns to the imaging from the original presentation of the patient.
- A resection of the primary tumor is then performed, taking the original imaging margins of the tumor into account.
- If the recurrence is large, the most recent imaging is used to guide the ablative procedure.
- Since these patients have been irradiated during the initial therapy, transfer of healthy, well-vascularized soft and/or hard tissue is an important component of the reconstruction.
- Regional and/or free flaps, which are commonly utilized during salvage procedures, are a critical part of the reconstructive ladder.
- This tissue can be used to reconstitute the primary organ involved (i.e., tongue, palate, mandible, pharynx) as well

as to cover and protect the carotid artery from exposure and/or salivary fistula.

▪ When a patient presents with a regional recurrence (i.e., within the cervical lymphatics), a cervical lymphadenectomy is performed in order to remove gross or microscopic disease within the neck.

▪ In the past, the radical neck dissection (extirpation of levels I–V with the accessory nerve, internal jugular vein, and sternocleidomastoid muscle) was performed routinely for all regional recurrences.

▪ Recently, the modified radical neck dissection (extirpation of levels I–V, preservation of the sternocleidomastoid muscle accessory nerve, and/or internal jugular vein) has been performed for regional recurrences.

▪ Although this was found to be significantly less morbid than the radical neck dissection, it still has its inherent complications (i.e., lymphedema, chronic shoulder pain, cosmetic deformity, etc.).

▪ Recently, many surgeons have been incorporating the selective neck dissection into their algorithm, reducing morbidity and the length of surgery.

▪ A selective neck dissection is the removal of selective cervical lymphatic levels with preservation of all other structures.

▪ Another approach addressing isolated regional recurrences is to perform a comprehensive neck dissection, intraoperative radiation therapy, and a pectoralis flap for carotid coverage.

▪ The neck dissection type is dictated by the structures involved with the recurrent disease.

▪ The use of the pectoralis major muscle flap is to prevent wound breakdown and carotid exposure. This approach is operator dependent and requires special expertise that is not widely available.

▪ Salvage Reirradiation

▪ The outcomes for patients who have failed previous radiation therapy and then treated with reirradiation therapy alone are poor.

- Salvage treatments incorporating reirradiation with chemotherapy have yielded a modest but significant chance for salvage in a small subset of patients.
- These regimens have consisted primarily of twice-a-day radiation programs delivered on a one week on, one week off schedule with concurrent chemotherapy.
- Chemotherapy regimens have consisted of paclitaxel (Taxol)/cisplatin, or hydroxyurea/5-fluorouracil.[12,13] Grade 4–5 toxicity is reported in 25–28% with on-treatment mortality rates of 8%.
- The efficacy of reirradiation has been confirmed in a multi-institutional prospective trial.
- Two-year survival rates of 15–26% are reported.
- Use of IMRT may improve outcomes.[14]
- Currently, this option is utilized primarily for patients who have good performance status but are not candidates for resection.
- The toxicity of reirradiation includes fistula formation; carotid artery blowout; osteoradionecrosis; and soft-tissue ulceration, including the mucosa.
- Grade 4–5 toxicity occurs in 15–25%.
- Several strategies to improve tolerance to external-beam radiation is to utilize intensity-modulated radiation to minimize dose to normal structures, hyperfractionation, and less toxic concurrent chemotherapy regimens.

■ Reirradiation with Salvage Surgery

- With the incorporation of salvage surgery with reirradiation, the chance for locoregional control and survival appears to double to 16–32%.
- However, a recent randomized control study showed improved locoregional control but no survival benefit with postoperative reirradiation with chemotherapy and worse acute and chronic toxicity.[15]
- To improve tolerance to external beam reirradiation, salvage surgery to remove previously irradiated normal tissue and radiation-resistant tumor is combined with reconstruction with unirradiated pedicled flaps.

- Brachytherapy and intraoperative radiation offer an important option to deliver radiation directly to the tumor bed without reirradiating excessive amounts of normal tissue.
- Brachytherapy may be performed with permanent seed implantation or temporary interstitial catheter placement.
- Intraoperative radiation is advantageous as it is delivered when the tumor bed can be visualized after resection of the tumor and with normal tissue maximally displaced or shielded.
- Brachytherapy and intraoperative radiotherapy are often combined with reconstruction with vascularized free flaps to ensure proper healing of the reirradiated bed.
- Additional external-beam radiation therapy may be delivered in this scenario as dictated by the adequacy of resection and the pathologic findings.
- Outcomes for brachytherapy and intraoperative radiotherapy are best if a gross total resection with negative margin is obtained.
- Local control can be obtained in 2/3 of cases treated with intraoperative radiotherapy and gross resection.
- Wound breakdown, fistula, carotid artery blowout, and osteoradionecrosis are significantly less common in comparison to patients undergoing reirradiation alone.

■ References

1. Colevas AD. Chemotherapy options for patients with metastatic or recurrent squamous cell carcinoma of the head and neck. *J Clin Oncol.* 2006;24(17):2644–2652.
2. Jacobs C, Lyman G, Velez-Garcia E, et al. A phase III randomized study comparing cisplatin and fluorouracil as single agents and in combination for advanced squamous cell carcinoma of the head and neck. *J Clin Oncol.* 1992;10(2):257–263.
3. Forastiere A, Metch B, Schuller D, et al. Randomized comparison of cisplatin plus fluorouracil and carboplatin plus fluorouracil versus methotrexate in advanced squamous cell carcinoma of the head and neck: a Southwest Oncology Group study. *J Clin Oncol.* 1992;10(8):1245–1251.
4. Vermorken J, Hitt R, Geoffrois L, et al. Cetuximab plus platinum-based therapy first-line in recurrent and/or metastatic (R/M) squamous cell carcinoma of the head and neck

(SCCHN): efficacy and safety results of a randomized phase III trial (EXTREME). *Eur J Cancer.* 2007;5:4(abstract No. 5501).

5. Posner MR, Hershock DM, Blajman CR, et al. Cisplatin and fluorouracil alone or with docetaxel in head and neck cancer. *N Engl J Med.* 2007;357(17):1705–1715.

6. Caponigro F, Massa E, Manzione L, et al. Docetaxel and cisplatin in locally advanced or metastatic squamous-cell carcinoma of the head and neck: a phase II study of the Southern Italy Cooperative Oncology Group (SICOG). *Ann Oncol.* 2001;12:199–202.

7. Schoffski P, Catimel G, Planting A, et al. Docetaxel and cisplatin: an active regimen in patients with locally advanced, recurrent, or metastatic squamous cell carcinoma of the head and neck. *Ann Oncol.* 1999;10(1):119–122.

8. Catimel G, Verwij J, Hanauske A. Docetaxel (Taxotere): an active drug for the treatment of patients with advanced squamous cell carcinoma of the head and neck. *Ann Oncol.* 1994;5:553–537.

9. Bonner JA, Harari PM, Giralt J, et al. Radiotherapy plus cetuximab for squamous-cell carcinoma of the head and neck. *N Engl J Med.* 2006;354(6):567–578.

10. Vermorken JB, Trigo J, Hitt R, et al. Open-label, uncontrolled, multicenter phase II study to evaluate the efficacy and toxicity of cetuximab as a single agent in patients with recurrent and/or metastatic squamous cell carcinoma of the head and neck who failed to respond to platinum-based therapy. *J Clin Oncol.* 2007;25(16):2171–2177.

11. Vermorken JB, Mesia R, Rivera F, et al. Platinum-based chemotherapy plus cetuximab in head and neck cancer. *N Engl J Med.* 2008;359(11):1116–1127.

12. Spencer SA, Harris J, Wheeler RH. Final report of RTOG 9610, a multi-institutional trial of reirradiation and chemotherapy for unresectable recurrent squamous cell carcinoma of the head and neck. *Int J Radiat Oncol Biol Phys.* 2006;64(2):382–391.

13. Langer CJ, Harris J, Horwitz EM. Phase II study of low-dose paclitaxel and cisplatin in combination with split-course concomitant twice-daily reirradiation in recurrent squamous cell carcinoma of the head and neck: results of Radiation Therapy Oncology Group Protocol 9911. *J Clin Oncol.* 2007;25(30):4800–4805.

14. Sulman EP, Schwartz DL, Le TT, et al. IMRT reirradiation of head and neck cancer-disease control and morbidity outcomes. *Int J Radiat Oncol Biol Phys.* 2009;73(2):399–409.

15. Janot F, de Raucourt D, Benhamou E. Randomized trial of postoperative reirradiation combined with chemotherapy after salvage surgery compared with salvage surgery alone in head and neck carcinoma. *J Clin Oncol.* 2008;26(34):5518–5523.

Head and Neck Reconstruction

■ Introduction

- Since the 1980s, head and neck reconstruction has evolved from simply patching a defect with a skin graft or rotated flap to a much more sophisticated attempt to restore both form and function.

- This shift in emphasis has occurred in synchronicity with the shift from the era of pedicled flaps to the era of free-tissue transfer.

- Surgeons can now transfer a wide variety of both hard and soft tissue in an efficient and reliable manner.

- Additionally, as a result of the advancements in reconstructive surgery, oncologic surgeons have been able to push the limits of ablative surgery, allowing for larger, more complex defects.

- The contemporary head and neck reconstructive team must be multidisciplinary in order to provide patients with the best possible outcome.

- The team should include a microvascular surgeon, an oral and maxillofacial surgeon, an oral and maxillofacial prosthodontist, an oculoplastic surgeon, and a speech and swallowing therapist.

- Since there is such a wide variety of local, regional, and free flaps that can be utilized to reconstruct a defect, the surgeon is no longer restricted in tissue availability, characteristics, or volume.

- Maxillofacial prosthetic planning represents an important consideration.

- The use of osseointegrated implants as part of this planning has become a key component in the final restoration of a patient's dental form and function.

- The following sections list of some of the commonly utilized regional and free flaps in head and neck reconstruction.

Regional Flaps

Pectoralis Major Flap

Figure 10.1 shows a pectoralis major flap.

- The pectoralis flap is a large myocutaneous flap that can be harvested quickly and is applied to a large variety of defects (i.e., pharynx, oral cavity, cutaneous defects).
- It is supplied by the pectoral artery and vein, which are branches of the thoracoacromial artery and vein.

Deltopectoral Flap

The deltopectoral flap (aka the Bakamjian flap) is a fasciocutaneous flap that is harvested based on the first, second, and third parasternal perforators.

Superior Trapezius Flap

The superior trapezius flap is a myocutaneous flap that is harvested based on the first, second, and third paraspinal perforators. This flap can be rotated to reach the ipsilateral neck.

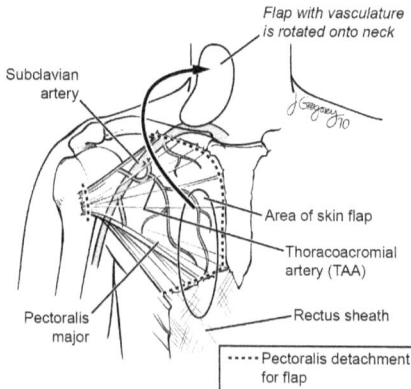

Figure 10.1 Pectoralis Major Flap
Source: Courtesy of Jill K. Gregory, Continuum Health Partners.

Latissimus Dorsi Flap

The latissimus dorsi flap is a very large myocutaneous flap that is based on the thoracoacromial artery and vein. This flap can be harvested as either a pedicled flap or a free flap.

■ Free Flaps

Radial Forearm Flap

Figure 10.2 shows a radial forearm flap.

- The radial forearm flap is most commonly harvested as a fasciocutaneous flap, although it can be harvested as an osseocutaneous flap (i.e., the radial bone).
- This flap is based on the radial artery and its vena comitantes.

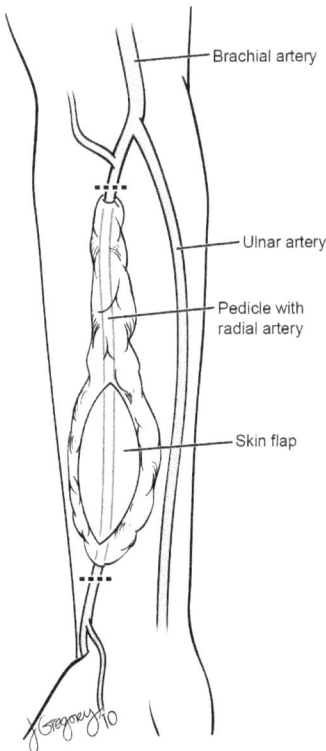

Figure 10.2 Radial Forearm Flap
Source: Courtesy of Jill K. Gregory, Continuum Health Partners.

- Often this flap is based on both the deep venous system (vena comitantes) and the superficial venous system (cephalic vein).
- It can be harvested with neural input from the medial antebrachial cutaneous nerve.
- This is the most common flap used to reconstruct large defects in the oral tongue or floor of the mouth as well the pharynx.

Anterolateral Thigh Flap

- The anterolateral thigh flap is most commonly harvested as a fasciocutaneous flap, although it can be harvested with muscle as well (vastus lateralis).
- This flap is based on the descending branch of the circumflex femoral artery and vein. It is usually harvested with little difficulty and results in very little morbidity to the patient.

Rectus Abdominis Flap

Figure 10.3 shows a rectus abdominis flap.

- The rectus abdominis flap is a very hardy myocutaneous flap that is based on the deep inferior epigastric artery and vein.

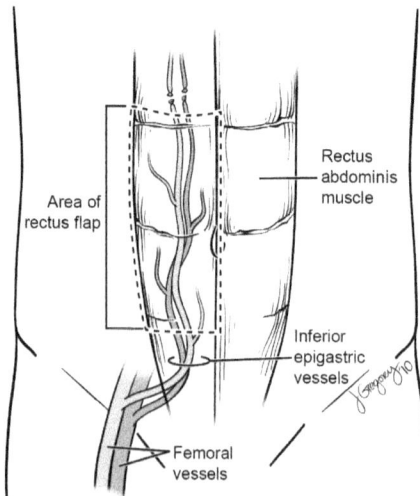

Figure 10.3 Rectus Abdominis Flap
Source: Courtesy of Jill K. Gregory, Continuum Health Partners.

▪ This flap provides the surgeon with a well-vascularized large-volume muscular flap that can be easily harvested in the supine position so that a two-team approach can be used.

Subscapular System

▪ The subscapular system provides a wide variety of different skin paddles (scapular and parascapular), bone (lateral border and tip of scapula), and muscle (latissimus), which can be harvested off of a single vascular pedicle.
▪ This flap can be used to reconstruct highly complex defects that demand a composite of material.

Fibular Free Flap

▪ The fibular free flap is a workhorse flap in head and neck reconstruction. This flap provides the longest segment of bone available.
▪ It has a thigh cortex, which makes it highly amenable to osseointegrated implants for dental rehabilitation. It is based on the peroneal artery and vein.

Iliac Crest Free Flap

▪ The iliac crest free flap is bone flap that provides very thick cortical bone, which is very amenable to osseointegrated implants.
▪ This flap is based on the deep circumflex iliac artery and vein. This flap can be harvested with internal oblique muscle.

▪ Mandible Reconstruction

The fibular free flap (**Figure 10.4**) is a workhorse flap in head and neck reconstruction. This flap provides the longest segment of bone available. It has a thigh cortex, which makes it highly amenable to osseointegrated implants for dental rehabilitation. It is based on the peroneal artery and vein.

The iliac crest free flap is bone flap (**Figure 10.5**) that provides very thick cortical bone, which is very amenable to osseointegrated implants. This flap is based on the deep

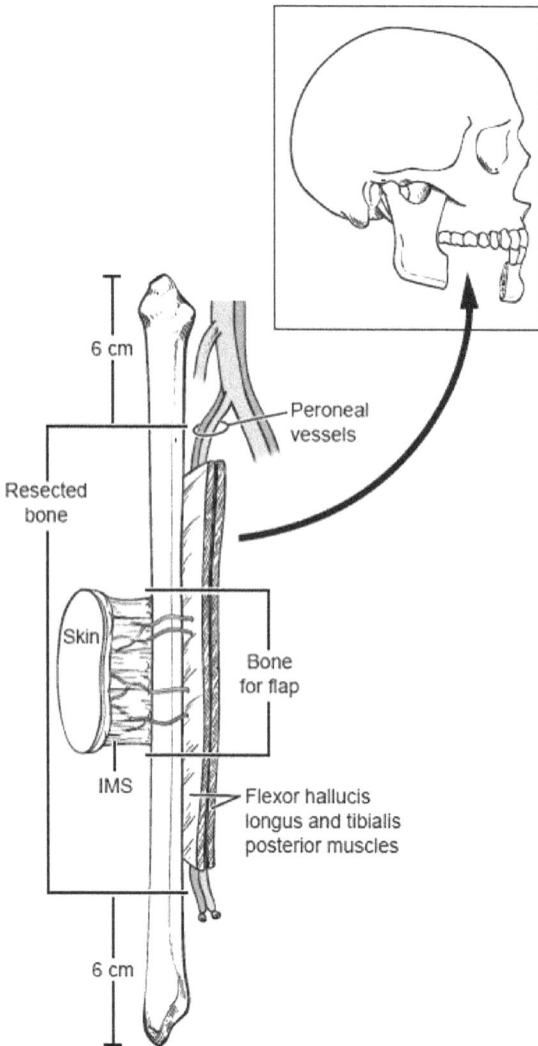

Figure 10.4 Fibular Free Flap
Source: Courtesy of Jill K. Gregory, Continuum Health Partners.

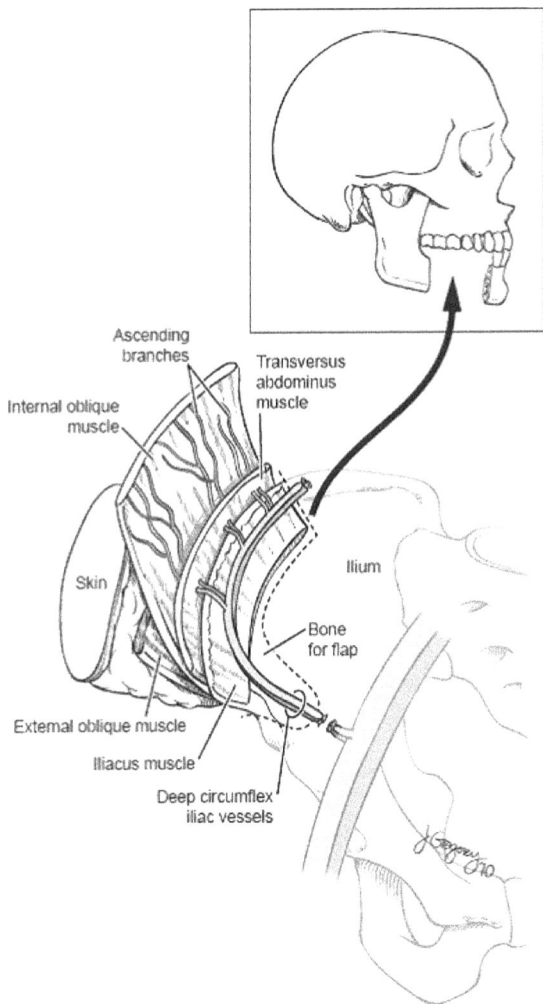

Figure 10.5 Iliac Crest Free Flap
Source: Courtesy of Jill K. Gregory, Continuum Health Partners.

circumflex iliac artery and vein. This flap can be harvested with internal oblique muscle.

The subscapular system (**Figure 10.6**) provides a wide variety of different skin paddles (scapular and parascapular), bone (lateral border and tip of scapula), and muscle (latissimus), which can be harvested off of a single vascular

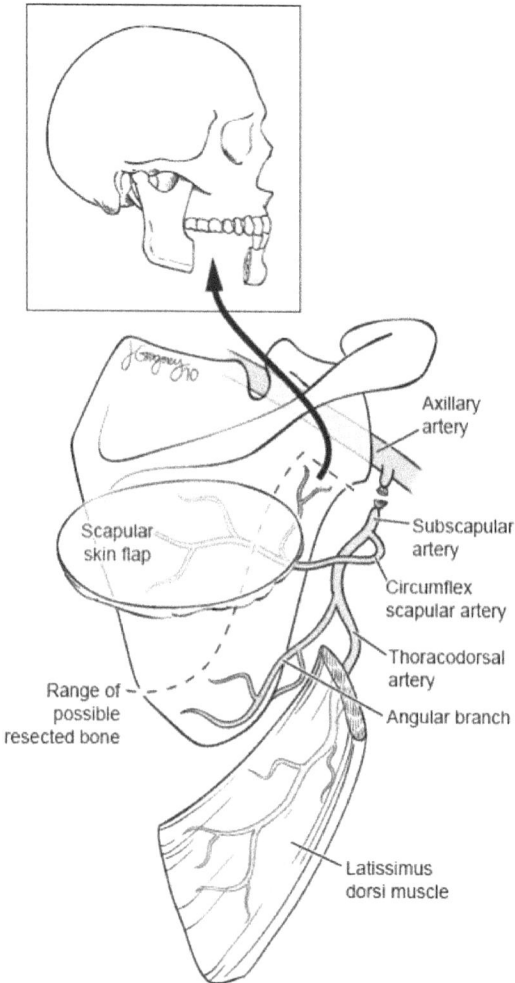

Figure 10.6 Subscapular System
Source: Courtesy of Jill K. Gregory, Continuum Health Partners.

pedicle. This flap can be used to reconstruct highly complex defects that demand a composite of material.

■ Pharyngeal Reconstruction

Figure 10.7 shows pectoralis flap reconstruction.

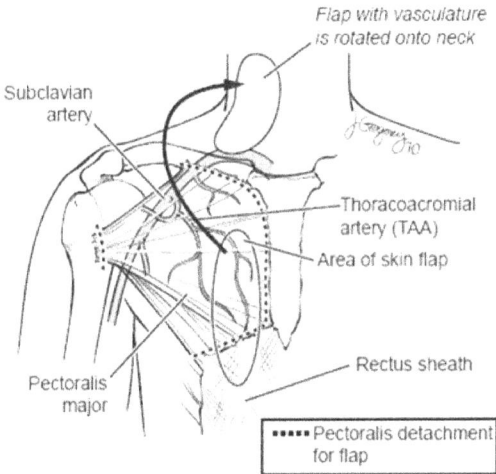

Figure 10.7 Pectoralis Flap Reconstruction
Source: Courtesy of Jill K. Gregory, Continuum Health Partners.

Index

Figures and tables are indicated by f and t following the page numbers.

www.ingramcontent.com/pod-product-compliance
Lightning Source LLC
Chambersburg PA
CBHW070736220326
41598CB00024BA/3448